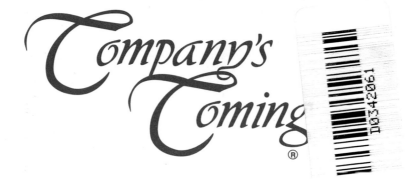

Diabetic Dinners

Jean Paré

www.companyscoming.com
visit our ↰ website

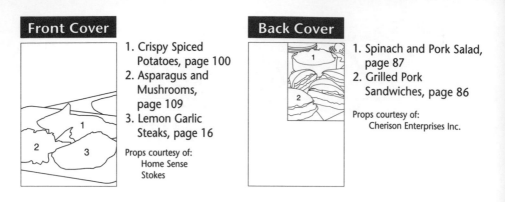

Front Cover

1. Crispy Spiced Potatoes, page 100
2. Asparagus and Mushrooms, page 109
3. Lemon Garlic Steaks, page 16

Props courtesy of:
Home Sense
Stokes

Back Cover

1. Spinach and Pork Salad, page 87
2. Grilled Pork Sandwiches, page 86

Props courtesy of:
Cherison Enterprises Inc.

Diabetic Dinners

Copyright © Company's Coming Publishing Limited

Sixth Printing September 2013

Library and Archives Canada Cataloguing in Publication
Paré, Jean, date-
Diabetic dinners / Jean Paré.
(Original series) Includes index.
At head of title: Company's Coming.
ISBN 978-1-897069-97-4
1. Diabetes--Diet therapy--Recipes. I. Title. II. Series: Paré, Jean, date- . Original series.
RC662.P37 2009   641.5'6314   C2009-900800-9

Published by
Company's Coming Publishing Limited
2311 – 96 Street
Edmonton, Alberta, Canada T6N 1G3
Tel: 780-450-6223   Fax: 780-450-1857
www.companyscoming.com

Company's Coming is a registered trademark owned by Company's Coming Publishing Limited

We acknowledge the financial support of the Government of Canada through the Canada Book Fund for our publishing activities.

Printed in China

We gratefully acknowledge the following suppliers for their generous support of our Test and Photography Kitchens:

Broil King Barbecues
Corelle®
Hamilton Beach® Canada
Lagostina®
Proctor Silex® Canada
Tupperware®

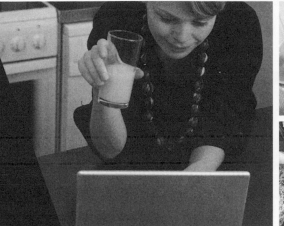
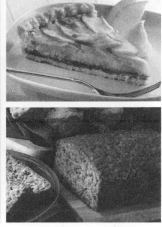

Company's Coming Cookbooks

Quick & easy recipes; everyday ingredients!

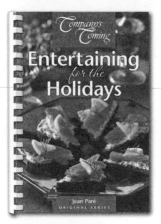

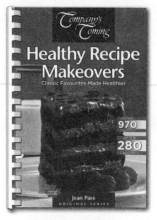

Original Series

- Softcover, 160 pages
- Lay-flat plastic comb binding
- Full-colour photos
- Nutrition information

Original Series

- Softcover, 160 pages
- Lay-flat plastic comb binding
- Full-colour photos
- Nutrition information

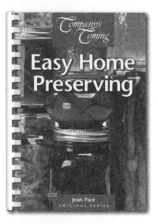

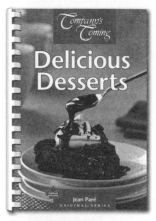

Original Series

- Softcover, 160 pages
- Lay-flat plastic comb binding
- Full-colour photos
- Nutrition information

Original Series

- Softcover, 160 pages
- Lay-flat plastic comb binding
- Full-colour photos
- Nutrition information

For a complete listing of our cookbooks, visit our website:
www.companyscoming.com

Table of Contents

Main Course
Dishes

Side Dishes

Condiments &
Sauces

Desserts

Snacks

The Company's Coming Story

Jean Paré (pronounced "jeen PAIR-ee") grew up understanding that the combination of family, friends and home cooking is the best recipe for a good life. From her mother, she learned to appreciate good cooking, while her father praised even her earliest attempts in the kitchen. When Jean left home, she took with her a love of cooking, many family recipes and an intriguing desire to read cookbooks as if they were novels!

"Never share a recipe you wouldn't use yourself."

When her four children had all reached school age, Jean volunteered to cater the 50th anniversary celebration of the Vermilion School of Agriculture, now Lakeland College, in Alberta, Canada. Working out of her home, Jean prepared a dinner for more than 1,000 people, launching a flourishing catering operation that continued for over 18 years. During that time, she had countless opportunities to test new ideas with immediate feedback—resulting in empty plates and contented customers! Whether preparing cocktail sandwiches for a house party or serving a hot meal for 1,500 people, Jean Paré earned a reputation for great food, courteous service and reasonable prices.

As requests for her recipes increased, Jean was often asked the question, "Why don't you write a cookbook?" Jean responded by teaming up with her son, Grant Lovig, in the fall of 1980 to form Company's Coming Publishing Limited. The publication of *150 Delicious Squares* on April 14, 1981 marked the debut of what would soon become one of the world's most popular cookbook series.

The company has grown since those early days when Jean worked from a spare bedroom in her home. Nowadays every Company's Coming recipe is *kitchen-tested* before it is approved for publication.

Company's Coming cookbooks are distributed in Canada, the United States, Australia and other world markets. Bestsellers many times over in English, Company's Coming cookbooks have also been published in French and Spanish.

Familiar and trusted in home kitchens around the world, Company's Coming cookbooks are offered in a variety of formats. Highly regarded as kitchen workbooks, the softcover Original Series, with its lay-flat plastic comb binding, is still a favourite among readers.

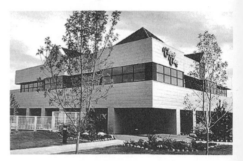

Jean Paré's approach to cooking has always called for *quick and easy recipes* using *everyday ingredients.* That view has served her well. The recipient of many awards, including the Queen Elizabeth Golden Jubilee Medal, Jean was appointed Member of the Order of Canada, her country's highest lifetime achievement honour.

Jean continues to share what she calls The Golden Rule of Cooking: *Never share a recipe you wouldn't use yourself.* It's an approach that has worked—*millions of times over!*

Foreword

Everyone with diabetes knows the importance of meal planning and eating the right foods. The delicious recipes in *Diabetic Dinners* are designed to be quick and easy to prepare, while helping to meet individual nutrition requirements.

Proper nutrition is the cornerstone for effective diabetes management. What, when and how much you eat are all critical factors in maintaining blood glucose levels. For this reason, *Diabetic Dinners* includes recipes lower in fat, sugar and sodium, as well as higher in fibre. For your assistance, detailed Nutrition Information, as well as meal-planning Choices, accompany each recipe. For more in-depth information on how we approached recipe development, read "The Recipes in this Cookbook," page 10.

Because eating timely meals is such a challenge, we've included several great snacks that fit within the parameters of most diabetics' needs. Toss several individual snack portions into your purse or into your child's backpack when on the go.

For those with a child who has diabetes, or for those who cook diabetic meals for the entire family, we've designed Kid-Friendly variations for many of the recipes. These variations cater to children's preferences and tastes. Preparing diabetic meals that are appropriate for everyone has never been easier!

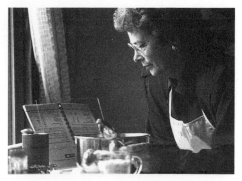

A healthy lifestyle, involving plenty of physical activity and balanced meals, is so important when living with diabetes. It takes a great deal of planning to regulate these aspects of your life. That's why we've tried to simplify the task of preparing healthy meals. Our recipes call for common ingredients, saving you time, energy and money.

Make mealtime more interesting with *Diabetic Dinners*—and remember that a healthy eating plan can include your favourite foods. Enjoy the wonderful variety of fresh flavours in this collection of healthy recipes your whole family will enjoy.

Jean Paré

Nutrition Information Guidelines

Each recipe is analyzed using the most current version of the Canadian Nutrient File from Health Canada, which is based on the United States Department of Agriculture (USDA) Nutrient Database.

- If more than one ingredient is listed (such as "butter or hard margarine"), or if a range is given (1 – 2 tsp., 5 – 10 mL), only the first ingredient or first amount is analyzed.
- For meat, poultry and fish, the serving size per person is based on the recommended 4 oz. (113 g) uncooked weight (without bone), which is 2 – 3 oz. (57 – 85 g) cooked weight (without bone)—approximately the size of a deck of playing cards.
- Milk used is 1% M.F. (milk fat), unless otherwise stated.

- Cooking oil used is canola oil, unless otherwise stated.
- Ingredients indicating "sprinkle," "optional," or "for garnish" are not included in the nutrition information.
- The fat in recipes and combination foods can vary greatly depending on the sources and types of fats used in each specific ingredient. For these reasons, the amount of saturated, monounsaturated and polyunsaturated fats may not add up to the total fat content.

Vera C. Mazurak, Ph.D.
Nutritionist

About Diabetes

Diabetes is a disease in which blood sugar (glucose) is not processed efficiently by the body due to the lack of insulin or insensitivity to insulin. Insulin is refined to process blood sugar into energy, otherwise it results in high glucose levels in the blood. Glucose levels are affected by digestion of carbohydrates, such as those found in grains, fruits and vegetables and milk, as well as in sugars, and by the production of glucose in the liver.

Prior to treatment, symptoms of diabetes may include increased thirst and urination, fatigue, vision changes and weight loss. Untreated, diabetes can damage the eyes, kidneys, nerves, heart and circulation system. Being physically active and maintaining a healthy body weight are keys to good living for everyone, but they are critical for those with diabetes.

In a healthy body, the pancreas produces enough insulin to enable glucose to enter cells and be used as energy. People with Type 1 diabetes have a severe lack of insulin because their pancreas produces little or none at all. In order to maintain normal blood sugar levels, many need to take insulin injections and to balance nutritional intake with activity. People with Type 2 diabetes don't produce enough insulin, or their bodies do not use it effectively. They may be able to manage the disease by weight management with diet and exercise alone, or with a combination of diet, exercise, and pills or insulin injections.

Diabetic Dinners is a cookbook filled with enticing, easy-to-prepare recipes. It follows dietary guidelines that are essentially the same for everyone—include more high-fibre, whole-grain products, and fruits and vegetables; and choose low-fat dairy products and leaner meats. People with diabetes need to consult with a registered dietitian to determine their best personal meal plan.

Most foods can be part of a diabetic meal plan. It is important to remember that some foods are more nutritious than others and therefore healthier and less damaging to our body. Alcohol, salt, fat, sugar and caffeine should be limited, but they don't necessarily need to be eliminated. Just like putting the wrong kind of gasoline in your car affects its performance, fuelling your body with poor food choices will do the same thing.

The cost of eating "premium fuel" doesn't have to be a premium price. For example, some cuts of meat may seem pricey, but they're not when you consider that a healthy portion of steak is 4 oz. (113 g) rather than the overly large 8 oz. (225 g) portion you are likely to get at a restaurant. Likewise, fresh fruits and vegetables fluctuate in price, so buy them in season and then compare the cost to their processed cousins-in-a-can. Be aware of convenience foods that are often high in fat, salt and sugar. Learn to read labels carefully.

Much has been said about how carbohydrates in starchy foods and refined sugars cause blood sugars to rise. But "carbs" still need to be part of a balanced, healthy diet. Carbohydrates with fibre (generally foods which have not been highly processed, such as fruits, vegetables, beans and whole-grain products) are more nutritious and better at maintaining even blood sugar levels than those from refined foods or sugars.

Advice about sugar consumption for people with diabetes has changed over the years. Small quantities of sugar distributed in foods throughout the day are now acceptable in a healthy eating plan because, in most people, blood sugar levels do not peak quickly. Up to 10% of total daily energy intake can come from sugar or added sugar in foods. For example, an 1800 calorie meal plan can include up to 180 calories from sugar, which is equivalent to 3 tbsp. (50 mL) of total sugar added to foods (e.g., jam, cranberry cocktail, regular soft drinks, cakes or desserts, chocolates, etc.).

Diabetic Choices (Beyond the Basics)

Tracking what you're eating is imperative for a diabetic diet. Each recipe includes a basic breakdown of nutritional information, as well as diabetic choice values for the Beyond the Basics meal-planning guide. Beyond the Basics groups together foods that are similar in carbohydrate content. The names of the categories have been changed to better reflect the foods in the group. For example, Starches has become Grains and Starches, whereas Sugars has become Other Choices to better reflect the sweets and snack foods within this group. Although the serving size of each food within a particular group may vary, one serving of each food in that group will have the same approximate composition of carbohydrates, protein, fat and calories. If no choices are listed, it means that the serving size suggested for that recipe does not contain enough carbohydrates to constitute a choice in any category.

For people on insulin who require precise carbohydrate counting, the nutritional information provides a useful guideline for total grams of carbohydrate and dietary fibre.

Nutrition Information

The Nutrition Information provided for each recipe in *Diabetic Dinners* tallies the calories, fat (including mono- and poly-unsaturated and saturated fats), cholesterol, carbohydrate, protein, fibre and sodium. These values include all ingredients listed in the recipe except those listed as "optional" or as a "garnish." If a range of measurements is given for an ingredient, the smaller amount is analyzed. There are also Kid-Friendly Ideas given at the end of selected recipes. The Nutrition Information and Choices are provided for these if there is a significant difference from those given for the original recipe.

The Recipes in this Cookbook

- **Artificial Sweeteners:** We did not use artificial sweeteners at the request of our Focus Group.

- **Cheese:** In order to lower fat content but to maintain taste, we used light, sharp (old) Cheddar cheese, part-skim mozzarella and grated, light Parmesan cheese product. We did use grated fresh Parmesan cheese, however, when flavour needed to be enhanced in selected recipes.

- **Fats:** We used canola or olive oil instead of margarine where possible. In some recipes, margarine or butter was better for taste, but the amount was limited. Butter should be used in moderation since it is animal fat and contains cholesterol. All fats and oils contain 9 calories per gram (compared to 4 calories per gram for carbohydrates), but vegetable or olive oil is better for your arteries when used moderately. Where possible, non-stick cookware or cooking spray was used to reduce the fats and oils used.

- **Meats:** In testing these recipes, we trimmed all visible fat from meats prior to cooking. We also chose leaner cuts of meat, such as boneless, skinless chicken breast halves or beef sirloin.

- **Milk:** We used 1% milk, unless otherwise specified, because it is a commonly acceptable low-fat milk with essentially the same nutritional values as 2% or whole milk, except fat content.

- **Yogurt:** We used non-fat plain or flavoured yogurt. Remember, when heated, non-fat yogurt will be runny. Use low-fat yogurt instead if heating.

- **Cooking Methods:** We recommend baking, grilling, steaming, poaching and stir-frying to reduce the amount of fat needed to cook an item and to retain more of the nutrients in the food. Also, drain off fat whenever possible while cooking.

If you have any questions about how these recipes, or any other foods, can fit into the diet of someone with diabetes, please talk with your doctor or dietitian.

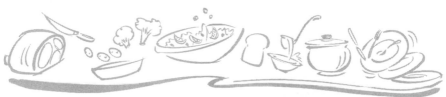

Beef and Mandarin Salad

This colourful, fresh salad is sure to get the taste buds jumping.

Lean beef inside round steak, trimmed of fat	12 oz.	340 g
Garlic salt	1/2 tsp.	2 mL
Can of unsweetened mandarin orange segments, drained	10 oz.	284 mL
Bag of mixed salad greens	6 cups	1.5 L
Thinly sliced red onion	1/2 cup	125 mL
Thinly sliced red pepper	1/2 cup	125 mL
PARMESAN DRESSING		
Finely grated fresh Parmesan cheese	2 tbsp.	30 mL
Olive oil	2 tbsp.	30 mL
Lemon juice	2 tbsp.	30 mL
Liquid honey	2 tsp.	10 mL
Garlic clove, minced (or 1/4 tsp., 1 mL, powder)	1	1
Pepper	1/4 tsp.	1 mL

Sprinkle steak with garlic salt. Preheat electric grill for 5 minutes or gas barbecue to medium-high. Cook steak on greased grill for about 5 minutes per side until desired doneness. Remove from heat. Let stand for 10 minutes. Slice into 1/4 inch (6 mm) thick strips.

Combine next 4 ingredients in large bowl. Add beef. Toss.

Parmesan Dressing: Combine all 6 ingredients in jar with tight-fitting lid. Shake well. Makes 1/3 cup (75 mL) dressing. Drizzle over salad. Toss gently. Makes 6 cups (1.5 L). Serves 4.

1 serving: 259 Calories; 13.4 g Total Fat (7.0 g Mono, 1.4 g Poly, 3.6 g Sat); 54 mg Cholesterol; 15 g Carbohydrate; 3 g Fibre; 21 g Protein; 245 mg Sodium

CHOICES: 1/2 Fruits; 3 Meat & Alternatives; 1 Fats

Apple Curry Wraps

*The unique combination of mild curry and a sweet apple tang will
tantalize your taste buds. Use different flavours of tortillas for variety.*

Olive oil	2 tsp.	10 mL
Beef sirloin steak, cut across grain into 1/8 inch (3 mm) thick slices	1/2 lb.	225 g
Chopped onion	1/4 cup	60 mL
Garlic cloves, minced (or 1/2 tsp., 2 mL, powder)	2	2
Mild green curry paste	1 1/2 tsp.	7 mL
Apple juice	1/3 cup	75 mL
Frozen peas, thawed	3/4 cup	175 mL
Medium peeled cooking apple (such as McIntosh), diced	1	1
Non-fat plain yogurt	1/2 cup	125 mL
Hot cooked short grain brown rice (about 1/2 cup, 125 mL, uncooked)	1 1/3 cups	325 mL
Flour tortillas (10 inch, 25 cm, diameter), warmed (see Tip, page 15)	4	4

Heat wok or large non-stick frying pan on medium until very hot. Add olive
oil. Add next 3 ingredients. Stir-fry for about 3 minutes until beef is no
longer pink inside and onion is softened.

Add curry paste and apple juice. Heat and stir until boiling.

Add peas and apple. Stir. Boil gently, uncovered, for about 1 minute until
heated through. Remove from heat.

Add yogurt. Stir.

Spoon rice along centre of each tortilla. Spoon beef mixture over rice. Fold
in sides. Roll up from bottom to enclose filling. Makes 4 wraps.

*1 wrap: 514 Calories; 14.9 g Total Fat (6.9 g Mono, 1.7 g Poly, 4.2 g Sat); 31 mg Cholesterol;
72 g Carbohydrate; 6 g Fibre; 23 g Protein; 618 mg Sodium*

CHOICES: 3 Grains & Starches; 1/2 Fruits; 1 1/2 Meat & Alternatives; 1/2 Fats

(continued on next page)

Kid-Friendly Idea: Omit curry paste. Substitute same amount of cooked long grain white rice for the brown.

1 wrap: 512 Calories; 14.2 g Total Fat (7.0 g Mono, 1.8 g Poly, 4.1 g Sat); 31 mg Cholesterol; 73 g Carbohydrate; 5 g Fibre; 23 g Protein; 552 mg Sodium

CHOICES: 3 1/2 Grains & Starches; 1/2 Fruits; 1 Vegetables; 1 1/2 Meat & Alternatives; 1/2 Fats

Mushroom Beef Burgers

A hearty and tasty make-ahead meal that everyone will love.

Canola oil	1 tbsp.	15 mL
Thinly sliced onion	1 cup	250 mL
Sliced fresh white mushrooms	2 cups	500 mL
Seasoned salt	1/4 tsp.	1 mL
Extra-lean ground beef	1 lb.	454 g
Finely chopped onion	1/2 cup	125 mL
Finely chopped fresh parsley	3 tbsp.	50 mL
(or 2 1/4 tsp., 11 mL, flakes)		
Barbecue sauce	2 tbsp.	30 mL
Pepper	1/4 tsp.	1 mL
Salsa	1/2 cup	125 mL
Hamburger buns, split, lightly toasted	4	4
Large tomato, sliced	1	1
Thinly sliced English cucumber (with peel)	1/2 cup	125 mL

Heat canola oil in large non-stick frying pan on medium. Add onion. Cook for 5 to 10 minutes, stirring occasionally, until onion is softened.

Add mushrooms and seasoned salt. Cook on medium-high for about 5 minutes, stirring occasionally, until mushrooms begin to brown.

Combine next 5 ingredients in large bowl. Shape into 4 patties. Preheat electric grill for 5 minutes or gas barbecue to medium. Cook patties on greased grill for about 5 minutes per side until no longer pink inside.

Spread salsa on both sides of each bun. Layer patty, mushroom mixture, tomato and cucumber, in order given, on bottom half of each bun. Cover with top halves. Makes 4 burgers.

1 burger: 329 Calories; 10.2 g Total Fat (4.6 g Mono, 2.5 g Poly, 2.3 g Sat); 60 mg Cholesterol; 31 g Carbohydrate; 2 g Fibre; 28 g Protein; 545 mg Sodium

CHOICES: 1 1/2 Grains & Starches; 1 Vegetables; 3 Meat & Alternatives; 1/2 Fats

Beef and Asparagus

Fresh, tender-crisp vegetables and beef are so good in an Asian-influenced sauce. Sprinkles of sesame seeds dress up this colourful dish. Serve with steamed broccoli and brown or white rice.

Dry sherry	1 tbsp.	15 mL
Low-sodium soy sauce	1 tbsp.	15 mL
Sesame oil	1 tsp.	5 mL
Garlic cloves, minced	2	2
(or 1/2 tsp., 2 mL, powder)		
Finely grated ginger root	1/2 tsp.	2 mL
Beef sirloin steak, cut across grain into 1/8 inch (3 mm) by 2 inch (5 cm) strips	1 lb.	454 g
Low-sodium prepared beef broth	1/3 cup	75 mL
Cornstarch	2 tsp.	10 mL
Low-sodium soy sauce	2 tbsp.	30 mL
Sweet chili sauce	1 tbsp.	15 mL
Canola oil	2 tsp.	10 mL
Canola oil	2 tsp.	10 mL
Fresh asparagus, trimmed of tough ends and cut into 2 inch (5 cm) pieces	12 oz.	340 g
Small cauliflower florets	1 cup	250 mL
Small onion, cut lengthwise into 6 wedges	1	1
Slivered red pepper	1/2 cup	125 mL
Sesame seeds, toasted (see Tip, page 97)	1 tsp.	5 mL

Combine first 5 ingredients in medium bowl.

Add beef to sherry mixture. Stir until coated. Cover. Marinate at room temperature for 15 minutes.

Stir broth into cornstarch in small cup until smooth. Add second amount of soy sauce and chili sauce. Stir. Set aside.

(continued on next page)

Heat wok or large non-stick frying pan on medium-high until very hot. Add first amount of canola oil. Add beef mixture. Stir-fry for 2 minutes. Transfer to plate.

Add second amount of canola oil to same wok. Add next 4 ingredients. Stir-fry for 3 to 4 minutes until asparagus is bright green and tender-crisp. Add beef mixture. Stir cornstarch mixture. Add to beef mixture. Heat and stir for about 1 minute until boiling and thickened.

Sprinkle with sesame seeds. Makes 4 cups (1 L). Serves 4.

1 serving: 321 Calories; 18.1 g Total Fat (7.6 g Mono, 1.9 g Poly, 5.2 g Sat); 61 mg Cholesterol; 14 g Carbohydrate; 4 g Fibre; 26 g Protein; 506 mg Sodium

CHOICES: 1 Vegetables; 3 Meat & Alternatives; 1 Fats

Pictured on page 17.

Kid-Friendly Idea: Substitute ketchup for the chili sauce. Substitute kid-friendly vegetables like carrots and sugar snap peas for the asparagus, cauliflower, onion and/or red pepper.

1 serving: 354 Calories; 18.1 g Total Fat (7.6 g Mono, 1.9 g Poly, 5.1 g Sat); 61 mg Cholesterol; 20 g Carbohydrate; 5 g Fibre; 26 g Protein; 545 mg Sodium

CHOICES: 3 Vegetables; 3 Meat & Alternatives

Paré Pointer

Actually, elephants have ivory tusks because iron ones would rust.

 To warm tortillas, wrap in foil or damp tea towel and heat in 200°F (95°C) oven for 10 minutes. Or sprinkle individual tortillas with water. Microwave, 1 or 2 at a time, on high (100%) for 20 seconds.

Lemon Garlic Steaks

A good recipe to make ahead. The lemon juice adds a fresh zing to the marinade. Serve with a fresh garden salad and cooked mushrooms.

Chopped fresh parsley	1/4 cup	60 mL
Lemon juice	3 tbsp.	50 mL
Sweet chili sauce	2 tbsp.	30 mL
Olive oil	1 tbsp.	15 mL
Garlic cloves, minced	2	2
(or 1/2 tsp., 2 mL, powder)		
Pepper	1 tsp.	5 mL
Beef strip loin steaks, trimmed of fat and cut into 4 pieces	1 lb.	454 g

Combine first 6 ingredients in medium bowl.

Add steak. Turn until coated. Cover. Marinate in refrigerator for at least 8 hours or overnight. Drain and discard marinade. Preheat electric grill for 5 minutes or gas barbecue to medium-high. Cook steak on greased grill for about 5 minutes per side until desired doneness. Serves 4.

1 serving: 199 Calories; 9.6 g Total Fat (4.4 g Mono, 0.5 g Poly, 3.3 g Sat); 58 mg Cholesterol; 3 g Carbohydrate; trace Fibre; 24 g Protein; 84 mg Sodium

CHOICES: 3 1/2 Meat & Alternatives

Pictured on front cover and on page 89.

Kid-Friendly Idea: Omit the garlic and use only 1/4 tsp. (1 mL) pepper.

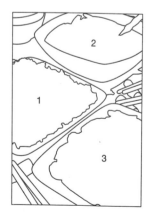

1. Fried Rice, page 98
2. Asian Citrus Chicken, page 22
3. Beef and Asparagus, page 14

Props courtesy of: Cherison Enterprises Inc.
Island Pottery Inc.

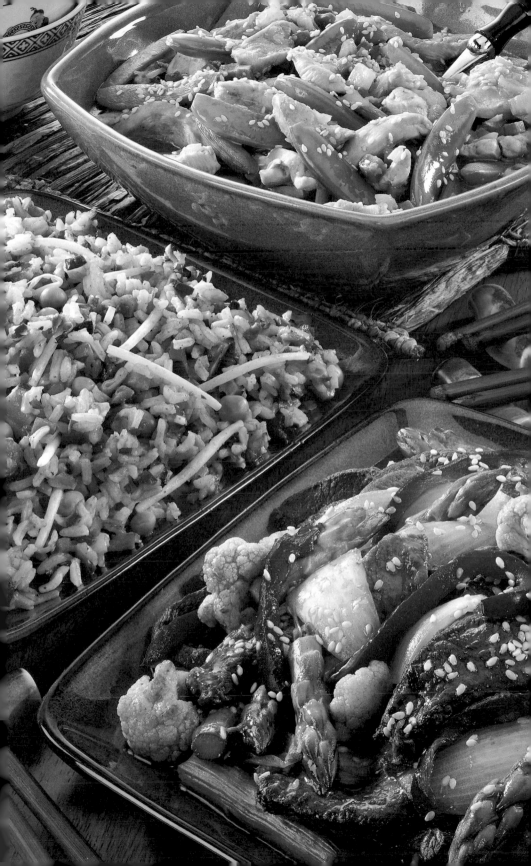

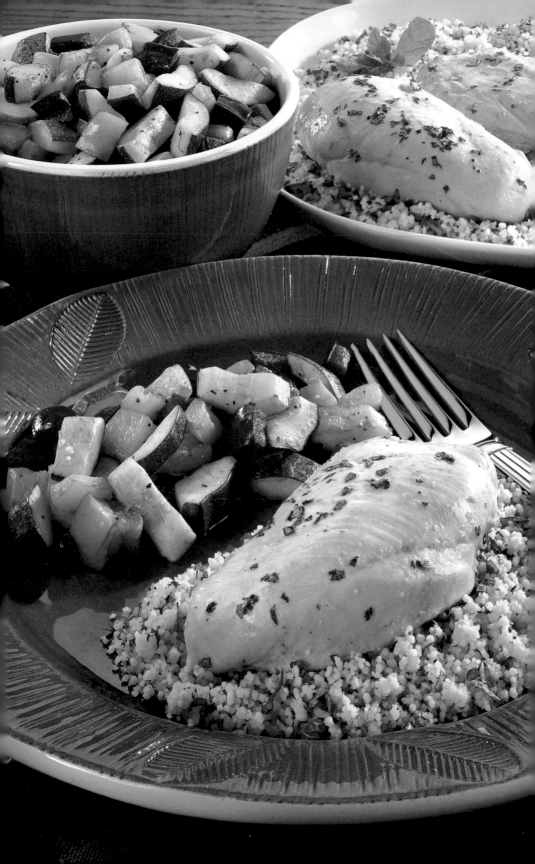

Pineapple Chicken Balls

Chicken, pineapple and green pepper in a sweet-and-sour sauce that's perfect over hot rice.

Large egg	1	1
Sliced green onion	1/4 cup	60 mL
Quick-cooking rolled oats	1/2 cup	125 mL
Low-sodium chicken bouillon powder	1 tsp.	5 mL
Dried thyme	1/4 tsp.	1 mL
Lean ground chicken	1 lb.	454 g
Can of pineapple tidbits (with juice)	14 oz.	398 mL
White vinegar	3 tbsp.	50 mL
Brown sugar, packed	2 tbsp.	30 mL
Low-sodium soy sauce	2 tbsp.	30 mL
Medium green pepper, diced	1	1
Water	3 tbsp.	50 mL
Cornstarch	1 1/2 tbsp.	25 mL

Combine first 5 ingredients in medium bowl.

Add chicken. Mix well. Shape into about forty 1 inch (2.5 cm) balls. Arrange in single layer on greased baking sheet with sides. Bake, uncovered, in 400°F (205°C) oven for about 15 minutes until browned and no longer pink inside.

Combine next 5 ingredients in large frying pan. Heat on medium-high, stirring occasionally, until boiling. Reduce heat to medium-low. Cover. Boil gently for 3 minutes.

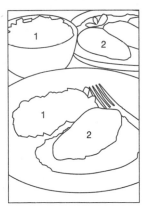

Stir water into cornstarch in small dish until smooth. Add to pineapple mixture. Heat and stir until boiling and thickened. Add meatballs. Stir. Heat, stirring occasionally, for 5 minutes. Serves 4.

1 serving: 306 Calories; 11.0 g Total Fat (trace Mono, trace Poly, 2.9 g Sat); 129 mg Cholesterol; 33 g Carbohydrate; 3 g Fibre; 22 g Protein; 361 mg Sodium

CHOICES: 1/2 Grains & Starches; 1 Fruits; 2 1/2 Meats & Alternatives

1. Zucchini Pepper Combo, page 105
2. Poached Spice Chicken, page 26

Props courtesy of: Pfaltzgraff Canada

Chili Turkey Burgers

Hearty burgers that are great broiled or grilled. They have a tender texture and a spicy bite.

Lean ground turkey	3/4 lb.	340 g
Egg whites (large)	2	2
Medium jalapeño pepper (see Tip, page 113), finely diced	1	1
Green onions, finely chopped	2	2
Garlic cloves, minced (or 1/2 tsp., 2 mL, powder)	2	2
Chili powder	1 tsp.	5 mL
Paprika	1 tsp.	5 mL
Garlic and herb no-salt seasoning	2 tsp.	10 mL
Pepper	1/4 tsp.	1 mL
Light Monterey Jack cheese, sliced	2 oz.	57 g
Whole-wheat hamburger buns, split and toasted	4	4
Fat-free salad dressing	1/4 cup	60 mL
Prepared mustard	2 tbsp.	30 mL
Salsa	1/4 cup	60 mL
Red onion slices	4	4
Lettuce leaves	4	4
Large tomato slices	4	4

Combine first 9 ingredients in medium bowl. Mix well. Shape into 4 patties about 4 inches (10 cm) in diameter. Broil on centre rack in oven for 4 to 5 minutes per side until juices run clear and patties are no longer pink inside.

Place cheese over patties to melt.

Spread bottom half of each bun with next 3 ingredients. Place 1 patty on each bottom half. Top with remaining 3 ingredients. Cover with top halves. Makes 4 burgers.

1 burger: 283 Calories; 6.6 g Total Fat (0.7 g Mono, 1.1 g Poly, 2.2 g Sat); 44 mg Cholesterol; 29 g Carbohydrate; 5 g Fibre; 31 g Protein; 551 mg Sodium

CHOICES: 1 Grains & Starches; 1/2 Vegetables; 3 1/2 Meat & Alternatives

Fish Parcels

Tender fish topped with tomato and fresh dill. The warm aroma will excite your senses.

Red snapper fillets, skin and any small bones removed, cut into 4 pieces	1 1/4 lbs.	560 g
Finely chopped tomato	1 cup	250 mL
Lemon juice	3 tbsp.	50 mL
Chopped fresh dill (or 3/4 tsp., 4 mL, dried)	1 tbsp.	15 mL
Olive oil	1 tbsp.	15 mL
Garlic salt	1/2 tsp.	2 mL
Pepper	1/4 tsp.	1 mL

Place each fish portion on greased 10 x 12 inch (25 x 30 cm) sheet of foil.

Combine remaining 6 ingredients in small bowl. Spoon over each portion of fish. Bring long sides of foil together. Fold over to form parcel. Fold short sides in to secure. Arrange parcels on ungreased baking sheet. Bake in 400°F (205°C) oven for 15 minutes. Carefully open parcel. Fish should flake easily when tested with fork. Serves 4.

1 serving: 183 Calories; 5.5 g Total Fat (2.9 g Mono, 1.2 g Poly, 0.9 g Sat); 52 mg Cholesterol, 3 g Carbohydrate; 1 g Fibre; 30 g Protein; 213 mg Sodium

CHOICES: 4 Meat & Alternatives; 1/2 Fats

Pictured on page 35.

 tip To make uniform-sized meatballs, use a small scoop. This looks like a miniature ice cream scoop and is available in various sizes at kitchen and restaurant supply stores. Or press meat mixture into a square or rectangle shape, same thickness all over. Cut into smaller squares of equal size. Roll each square into a ball.

Asian Citrus Chicken

Tender chicken and snap peas are so good in this orange sauce. Perfect served over rice.

Orange juice	3/4 cup	175 mL
Cornstarch	1 tbsp.	15 mL
Hoisin sauce	2 tbsp.	30 mL
Oyster sauce	1 tbsp.	15 mL
Rice vinegar	1 tbsp.	15 mL
Brown sugar, packed	2 tsp.	10 mL
Finely grated orange zest	1 tsp.	5 mL
Olive oil	2 tsp.	10 mL
Boneless, skinless chicken breast halves, cut into thin strips	3/4 lb.	340 g
Garlic cloves, minced (or 1/2 tsp., 2 mL, powder)	2	2
Ground ginger	1/2 tsp.	2 mL
Chopped onion	1 cup	250 mL
Chopped celery	1 cup	250 mL
Chopped carrot	2/3 cup	150 mL
Low-sodium prepared chicken broth	1/2 cup	125 mL
Sugar snap peas, trimmed	2 cups	500 mL
Sesame seeds, toasted (see Tip, page 97),	2 tsp.	10 mL

Stir orange juice into cornstarch in small bowl until smooth. Add next 5 ingredients. Stir. Set aside.

Heat wok or large non-stick frying pan on medium-high. Add olive oil. Add chicken. Add garlic and ginger. Stir-fry for about 4 minutes until chicken is no longer pink inside.

Add next 3 ingredients. Stir-fry for 2 minutes.

Add broth and peas. Stir. Reduce heat to medium. Cover. Boil gently for 3 to 5 minutes until carrot is tender-crisp and peas are bright green. Stir cornstarch mixture. Add to chicken mixture. Heat and stir until mixture is boiling and thickened.

Sprinkle with sesame seeds. Makes 6 cups (1.5 L). Serves 4.

1 serving: 235 Calories; 4.4 g Total Fat (2.0 g Mono, 0.7 g Poly, 0.7 g Sat); 50 mg Cholesterol; 26 g Carbohydrate; 3 g Fibre; 23 g Protein; 479 mg Sodium

CHOICES: 1/2 Fruits; 2 Vegetables; 1 Meat & Alternatives; 1/2 Fats

Pictured on page 17.

Blackened Snapper

The delicious spices on this tender fish are cooled down with a minty yogurt sauce. You may want to cook this on the barbecue to keep the household smoke detector from sounding.

All-purpose flour	2 tbsp.	30 mL
Parsley flakes	1 tbsp.	15 mL
Finely grated lemon zest	2 tsp.	10 mL
Paprika	2 tsp.	10 mL
Pepper	1 tsp.	5 mL
Garlic powder	3/4 tsp.	4 mL
Onion powder	3/4 tsp.	4 mL
Cayenne pepper	1/4 tsp.	1 mL
Snapper fillets, skin and any small bones removed	1 lb.	454 g
Canola oil	2 tbsp.	30 mL
COOL YOGURT SAUCE		
Non-fat plain yogurt	2/3 cup	150 mL
Chopped fresh mint leaves	1 tbsp.	15 mL

Combine first 8 ingredients in small dish.

Arrange fillets on large sheet of waxed paper. Sprinkle flour mixture over both sides of fillets. Press fillets into any loose mixture left on paper.

Heat large non-stick frying pan on medium-high until hot. Add 1 tbsp. (15 mL) canola oil. Tilt pan to coat. Add half of fillets. Cook for about 1 1/2 minutes per side until browned and fish flakes easily when tested with fork. Some smoking will occur. Transfer fish to plate. Keep warm. Repeat with remaining canola oil and fillets.

Cool Yogurt Sauce: Combine yogurt and mint in small bowl. Makes 2/3 cup (150 mL) sauce. Serve with fish. Serves 4.

1 serving: 215 Calories; 8.7 g Total Fat (4.3 g Mono, 2.6 g Poly, 0.9 g Sat); 43 mg Cholesterol; 8 g Carbohydrate; 1 g Fibre; 26 g Protein; 104 mg Sodium

CHOICES: 3 Meat & Alternatives

Kid-Friendly Idea: Omit cayenne pepper and reduce or omit pepper. Omit mint in the sauce.

Chicken and Pea Risotto

Parmesan cheese and mint enhance the flavour of this creamy risotto.
Peas add crispness.

Low-sodium prepared chicken broth	7 cups	1.75 L
Olive oil	2 tsp.	10 mL
Boneless, skinless chicken breast halves	1 lb.	454 g
Finely chopped onion	1 cup	250 mL
Garlic cloves, minced	2	2
(or 1/2 tsp., 2 mL, powder)		
Lemon pepper	1/2 tsp.	2 mL
Arborio rice	1 cup	250 mL
Long grain brown rice	1 cup	250 mL
Dry (or alcohol-free) white wine	1/2 cup	125 mL
Frozen peas	1 cup	250 mL
Chopped fresh basil	2 tbsp.	30 mL
(or 1 1/2 tsp., 7 mL, dried)		
Chopped fresh mint leaves	1 tbsp.	15 mL
(or 3/4 tsp., 4 mL, dried)		
Finely grated fresh Parmesan cheese	1/3 cup	75 mL

Bring broth to a boil in medium saucepan. Cover. Reduce to lowest heat.

Heat olive oil in large saucepan on medium-high. Add chicken. Cook for 6 to 8 minutes per side until well browned and no longer pink inside. Cut chicken into 1/2 inch (12 mm) pieces. Cover to keep warm.

Add next 3 ingredients to drippings in same saucepan. Heat and stir on medium for about 5 minutes, scraping any brown bits from bottom of saucepan, until onion is softened.

Add arborio rice and brown rice. Stir well.

Add wine. Heat and stir until wine is absorbed. Add warm broth, 1 cup (250 mL) at a time, stirring constantly until broth is absorbed. This will take about 30 minutes.

(continued on next page)

Add chicken and next 3 ingredients. Heat and stir until heated through.

Remove from heat. Add Parmesan cheese. Stir until melted. Makes 9 cups (2.25 L). Serves 6.

1 serving: 361 Calories; 5.6 g Total Fat (1.7 g Mono, 0.8 g Poly, 2.0 g Sat); 56 mg Cholesterol; 45 g Carbohydrate; 3 g Fibre; 28 g Protein; 918 mg Sodium

CHOICES: 2 Grains & Starches; 1 Vegetables; 3 Meat & Alternatives

---

Parmesan-Crumbed Fish

Snapper and sole work well in this recipe, but so will your favourite white fish.

Large egg	1	1
Milk	2 tsp.	10 mL
Fine dry bread crumbs	3/4 cup	175 mL
Finely grated fresh Parmesan cheese	3 tbsp.	50 mL
Chopped fresh parsley	3 tbsp.	50 mL
(or 2 1/4 tsp., 11 mL, flakes)		
Salt	1/4 tsp.	1 mL
All-purpose flour	3 tbsp.	50 mL
Snapper fillets, skin and any small bones removed, cut into 6 pieces	1 1/2 lbs.	680 g
Canola oil	1 1/2 tbsp.	25 mL

Beat egg and milk with fork in shallow dish.

Combine next 4 ingredients in separate shallow dish.

Measure flour onto sheet of waxed paper. Dredge fish in flour. Dip into egg mixture. Press into crumb mixture until coated.

Heat canola oil in large non-stick frying pan on medium. Add fish. Cook for about 3 minutes per side until fish is golden and flakes easily when tested with fork. Serves 6.

1 serving: 207 Calories; 6.8 g Total Fat (2.3 g Mono, 1.5 g Poly, 1.3 g Sat); 68 mg Cholesterol; 8 g Carbohydrate; trace Fibre; 27 g Protein; 290 mg Sodium

CHOICES: 1/2 Grains & Starches; 3 Meats & Alternatives; 1/2 Fats

Pictured on page 35.

To Make Ahead: Crumb fish. Cover. Chill for up to 4 hours.

Poached Spice Chicken

Lovely, moist chicken with a sweet and spicy sauce. Serve with Roasted Cauliflower, page 103, or Oven-Fried Vegetables, page 111.

SWEET AND SPICY SAUCE

Low-sodium prepared chicken broth	1 1/2 cups	375 mL
Orange juice	1 cup	250 mL
Dry (or alcohol-free) white wine	1/2 cup	125 mL
Liquid honey	2 tbsp.	30 mL
Whole green cardamom, bruised (see Tip, page 27)	6	6
Cinnamon stick (4 inch, 10 cm, length)	1	1
Ground cumin	1/2 tsp.	2 mL
Ground coriander	1/2 tsp.	2 mL
Chili powder	1/4 tsp.	1 mL
Boneless, skinless chicken breast halves (4 – 6 oz., 113 – 170 g, each)	4	4

HERB COUSCOUS

Low-sodium prepared chicken broth	3/4 cup	175 mL
Couscous	3/4 cup	175 mL
Olive oil	1 tsp.	5 mL
Chopped fresh mint leaves (or 1 1/2 tsp., 7 mL, dried)	2 tbsp.	30 mL
Chopped fresh cilantro (or fresh parsley)	2 tbsp.	30 mL

Sweet and Spicy Sauce: Combine first 9 ingredients in medium frying pan. Heat and stir on medium until boiling. Reduce heat to medium-low.

Add chicken. Cook, uncovered, for about 15 minutes, turning once, until chicken is no longer pink inside. Transfer chicken to 2 quart (2 L) casserole. Cover to keep warm. Boil cooking liquid on medium-high for about 15 minutes until reduced by half. Strain into small bowl, discarding solids. Makes about 1 1/3 cups (325 mL) sauce. Pour over chicken. Cover to keep warm.

(continued on next page)

Herb Couscous: Bring broth to a boil in medium saucepan. Remove from heat.

Add couscous and olive oil. Stir. Cover. Let stand for 5 minutes. Fluff with fork.

Add mint and cilantro. Stir. Makes 2 1/4 cups (550 mL) couscous. Serve with chicken and sauce. Serves 4.

1 serving: 303 Calories; 3.2 g Total Fat (1.2 g Mono, 0.5 g Poly, 0.6 g Sat); 69 mg Cholesterol; 33 g Carbohydrate; 1 g Fibre; 31 g Protein; 414 mg Sodium

CHOICES: 1 Grains & Starches; 1/2 Fruits; 1/2 Other Choices; 3 Meat & Alternatives

Pictured on page 18.

Kid-Friendly Idea: If children aren't used to the strong spices in this dish, they may not readily enjoy the flavour. Reduce spices the first time around to let kids gradually become familiar with the taste.

 To bruise cardamom, pound cardamom pods with a mallet or press with the flat side of a wide knife to "bruise" or crack them. Open slightly.

Creamy Fish Stew

Tender pieces of fish and baby clams are delicious in this creamy stew.
Asparagus and green beans add a splash of colour and a pleasing texture.

Hard margarine (or butter)	2 tsp.	10 mL
Finely chopped onion	1/2 cup	125 mL
All-purpose flour	2 tbsp.	30 mL
Dry (or alcohol-free) white wine	1/2 cup	125 mL
Milk	1 cup	250 mL
Low-sodium prepared chicken broth	1 cup	250 mL
Cod fillets, skin and any small bones removed, cut into 2 inch (5 cm) pieces	1 lb.	454 g
Fresh (or frozen, thawed) cut green beans	1 cup	250 mL
Fresh asparagus, trimmed of tough ends and cut into 1 inch (2.5 cm) pieces	1/2 lb.	225 g
Cans of whole baby clams (5 oz., 142 g, each), rinsed and drained	2	2
Chopped fresh dill (or 3/4 – 2 1/4 tsp., 4 – 11 mL, dried)	1 – 3 tbsp.	15 – 50 mL

Melt margarine in large pot or Dutch oven on medium. Add onion. Cook for 5 to 10 minutes, stirring often, until onion is softened.

Add flour. Heat and stir for 1 minute. Add next 3 ingredients. Heat and stir for about 5 minutes until boiling and thickened.

Add next 3 ingredients. Bring to a boil. Cover. Reduce heat to medium-low. Simmer for about 10 minutes, without stirring, until fish flakes easily when tested with fork and vegetables are tender-crisp.

Add clams and dill. Stir until heated through. Makes 6 3/4 cups (1.7 L). Serves 4.

1 serving: 278 Calories; 5.4 g Total Fat (0.4 g Mono, 0.3 g Poly, 1.6 g Sat); 110 mg Cholesterol; 16 g Carbohydrate; 2 g Fibre; 37 g Protein; 669 mg Sodium

CHOICES: 1 Vegetables; 4 1/2 Meats & Alternatives

Marinated Halibut Skewers

Flaky chunks of halibut with a generous sprinkling of dill. Great on the barbecue, too! Serve with Tropical Yogurt Topping, page 115, for a summertime feel.

Lime juice	2 tbsp.	30 mL
Dry (or alcohol-free) white wine	2 tbsp.	30 mL
Chopped fresh dill (or 3/4 tsp., 4 mL, dried)	1 tbsp.	15 mL
Garlic cloves, minced (or 1/4 – 1/2 tsp., 1 – 2 mL, powder)	1 – 2	1 – 2
Minced ginger root	1 tsp.	5 mL
Sesame oil	2 tsp.	10 mL
Halibut steaks, skin and any small bones removed, cut into 1 1/4 inch (3 cm) cubes	1 1/4 lbs.	560 g
Bamboo skewers (6 inch, 15 cm, length), soaked in water for 10 minutes	8	8

Combine first 6 ingredients in medium bowl.

Add fish. Stir until coated. Cover. Marinate in refrigerator for 1 hour. Stir. Remove fish. Discard marinade.

Thread 3 fish cubes, crosswise through grain of fish, close together onto each skewer. Place on greased wire rack set in broiler pan. Broil on top rack in oven for about 8 minutes, turning carefully at halftime, until fish flakes easily when tested with fork. Makes 8 skewers. Serves 4.

1 serving: 181 Calories; 5.6 g Total Fat (1.1 g Mono, 1.0 g Poly, 0.8 g Sat); 45 mg Cholesterol; 1 g Carbohydrate; trace Fibre; 30 g Protein; 77 mg Sodium

CHOICES: 4 Meat & Alternatives; 1/2 Fats

Kid-Friendly Idea: Use apple juice instead of white wine. You might also choose to omit ginger.

1 serving: 180 Calories; 5.6 g Total Fat (1.1 g Mono, 1.0 g Poly, 0.8 g Sat); 45 mg Cholesterol; 1 g Carbohydrate; trace Fibre; 30 g Protein; 77 mg Sodium

CHOICES: 4 Meat & Alternatives; 1/2 Fats

Variation: Preheat gas barbecue to medium. Place skewers on well-greased grill. Close lid. Cook for 6 to 8 minutes, turning carefully at halftime, until fish flakes easily when carefully tested with fork.

Chicken Mushroom Rolls

Thick, creamy cheese sauce covers pasta rolls flavoured with rosemary and thyme.

Boiling water	12 cups	3 L
Salt	1 tbsp.	15 mL
Whole-wheat lasagna noodles	10	10
CHICKEN MUSHROOM FILLING		
Olive oil	1 tsp.	5 mL
Lean ground chicken	1 lb.	454 g
Finely chopped onion	1/4 cup	60 mL
Garlic chili sauce	1 tsp.	5 mL
Finely chopped fresh white mushrooms	1 1/2 cups	375 mL
Finely chopped red pepper	1/3 cup	75 mL
Garlic and herb no-salt seasoning	1 tsp.	5 mL
Pepper	1/4 tsp.	1 mL
All-purpose flour	2 tbsp.	30 mL
Low-sodium prepared chicken broth	2/3 cup	150 mL
Finely chopped fresh thyme	1 tsp.	5 mL
(or 1/4 tsp., 1 mL, dried)		
Finely chopped fresh rosemary	1 tsp.	5 mL
(or 1/4 tsp., 1 mL, dried)		
PARMESAN CHEESE SAUCE		
Skim milk	2 cups	500 mL
All-purpose flour	2 tbsp.	30 mL
Finely grated fresh Parmesan cheese	1/4 cup	60 mL
Salt	1/4 tsp.	1 mL
Ground nutmeg	1/4 tsp.	1 mL

Combine boiling water and salt in large uncovered pot or Dutch oven. Add noodles. Cook, uncovered, for 10 to 12 minutes, stirring occasionally, until tender but firm. Drain. Rinse. Drain well.

Chicken Mushroom Filling: Heat olive oil in large non-stick frying pan on medium. Add next 3 ingredients. Scramble-fry for about 7 minutes until onion is softened and chicken is no longer pink.

(continued on next page)

Add next 4 ingredients. Cook, stirring often, until most liquid is evaporated.

Sprinkle with flour. Stir. Add next 3 ingredients. Heat and stir until boiling and thickened. Transfer to medium bowl. Let stand for about 15 minutes until cool. Spread 1/4 cup (60 mL) filling down length of each noodle. Roll up, jelly roll-style. Place rolls, seam-side down, in greased 9 x 13 inch (23 x 33 cm) pan.

Parmesan Cheese Sauce: Stir milk into flour in small saucepan until smooth. Heat and stir on medium for about 8 minutes until boiling and thickened.

Add remaining 3 ingredients. Stir. Pour over noodle rolls. Spread sauce evenly. Cover with greased foil. Bake in 350°F (175°C) oven for 30 minutes. Remove foil. Broil, uncovered, for about 10 minutes until bubbling and golden. Makes 10 rolls.

1 roll: 189 Calories; 5.4 g Total Fat (0.3 g Mono, 0.1 g Poly, 1.8 g Sat); 34 mg Cholesterol; 22 g Carbohydrate; 2 g Fibre; 14 g Protein; 218 mg Sodium

CHOICES: 1 Grains & Starches; 1 Meat & Alternatives

Kid-Friendly Idea: Substitute same amount of regular lasagna noodles for the whole wheat. Omit mushrooms and red pepper. Use 2 cups (500 mL) frozen mixed vegetables (thawed). Omit fresh herbs.

1 roll: 201 Calories; 5.4 g Total Fat (0.3 g Mono, 0.1 g Poly, 1.7 g Sat); 34 mg Cholesterol; 24 g Carbohydrate; 2 g Fibre; 14 g Protein; 227 mg Sodium

CHOICES: 1/2 Vegetables; 1 Meat & Alternatives

Lemon Asparagus Penne

This pasta has lots of fresh, lemony sauce for an exceptionally satisfying dish.

Boiling water	8 cups	2 L
Salt	2 tsp.	10 mL
Whole-wheat penne pasta	2 2/3 cups	650 mL
Part-skim ricotta cheese	3/4 cup	175 mL
Finely grated lemon zest	1 tbsp.	15 mL
Skim evaporated milk	1/2 cup	125 mL
Olive oil	1 tbsp.	15 mL
Fresh asparagus, trimmed of tough ends and cut into 1 inch (2.5 cm) pieces	1 1/2 lbs.	680 g
Garlic cloves, minced (or 3/4 tsp., 4 mL, powder)	3	3
Green onions, cut diagonally into 1 inch (2.5 cm) pieces	6	6
Finely grated fresh Parmesan cheese	2 tbsp.	30 mL

Combine boiling water and salt in large uncovered pot or Dutch oven. Add pasta. Boil, uncovered, for 10 to 12 minutes, stirring occasionally, until tender but firm. Drain, reserving 3/4 cup (175 mL) cooking water. Rinse pasta with hot water. Drain well. Return to pot.

Put ricotta cheese and lemon zest into blender or food processor. Add reserved hot cooking water and evaporated milk. Process until smooth.

Heat olive oil in large frying pan on medium. Add next 3 ingredients. Stir. Cover. Cook for about 5 minutes, shaking pan several times, until asparagus is tender-crisp and starting to brown. Add ricotta cheese mixture. Stir for about 2 minutes until heated through. Add to pasta. Toss. Transfer to serving bowl.

Sprinkle with Parmesan cheese. Makes 8 cups (2 L). Serves 4.

1 serving: 461 Calories; 11.4 g Total Fat (2.5 g Mono, 0.7 g Poly, 4.9 g Sat); 30 mg Cholesterol; 70 g Carbohydrate; 9 g Fibre; 23 g Protein; 290 mg Sodium

CHOICES: 3 Grains & Starches; 1 Vegetables; 1 Meat & Alternatives; 1/2 Fats

Shrimp and Asparagus Stir-Fry

Bright green asparagus lends crunch and flavour to this light, summery stir-fry. Serve this quick, easy-to-prepare dish with a bowl of steaming jasmine (or other) rice.

Low-sodium prepared chicken broth	1/4 cup	60 mL
Cornstarch	1 tsp.	5 mL
Low-sodium soy sauce	1 1/2 tbsp.	25 mL
Chili paste (sambal oelek)	1/2 tsp.	2 mL
Canola oil	2 tsp.	10 mL
Sliced green onion	1/3 cup	75 mL
Garlic cloves, minced	2	2
(or 1/2 tsp., 2 mL, powder)		
Finely grated ginger root	1 – 2 tsp.	5 – 10 mL
Medium uncooked shrimp, peeled and deveined	1 lb.	454 g
Fresh asparagus, trimmed of tough ends, cut into 1 inch (2.5 cm) pieces	1 lb.	454 g
Sesame seeds, toasted (see Tip, page 97)	1 tbsp.	15 mL

Stir broth into cornstarch in small dish until smooth. Add soy sauce and chili paste. Stir. Set aside.

Heat wok or large non-stick frying pan on medium-high until very hot. Add canola oil. Add next 3 ingredients. Stir-fry for 1 to 2 minutes until fragrant.

Add shrimp and asparagus. Stir cornstarch mixture. Add to shrimp mixture. Stir-fry for about 5 minutes until shrimp are pink and curled, asparagus is tender-crisp and sauce is thickened.

Sprinkle with sesame seeds. Makes 4 1/2 cups (1.1 L). Serves 4.

1 serving: 187 Calories; 5.5 g Total Fat (1.6 g Mono, 1.5 g Poly, 0.6 g Sat); 173 mg Cholesterol; 8 g Carbohydrate; 3 g Fibre; 27 g Protein; 425 mg Sodium

CHOICES: 3 Meats & Alternatives; 1/2 Fats

Pictured on page 35.

Maple Balsamic Tenderloin

Moist and perfectly cooked pork with sweet, tangy undertones. Great served with a salad and roasted potatoes.

Frozen concentrated apple juice, thawed	1/4 cup	60 mL
Maple syrup	1/4 cup	60 mL
Balsamic vinegar	3 tbsp.	50 mL
Garlic clove, minced	1	1
(or 1/4 tsp., 1 mL, powder)		
Pepper	1/4 tsp.	1 mL
Pork tenderloin, trimmed of fat	1 lb.	454 g

Combine first 5 ingredients in medium bowl.

Add pork. Turn until coated. Cover. Marinate in refrigerator for at least 8 hours or overnight, turning several times. Drain and discard marinade. Preheat gas barbecue to medium-high. Turn 1 burner off. Cook pork on greased grill on unlit side for 35 to 40 minutes, turning occasionally, until pork is tender and internal temperature reads 155°F (68°C). Remove to platter. Cover with foil. Let stand for 10 minutes. Internal temperature should rise to at least 160°F (70°C). Cut into 1 inch (2.5 cm) thick slices. Serves 4.

1 serving: 136 Calories; 3.9 g Total Fat (1.8 g Mono, 0.4 g Poly, 1.3 g Sat); 74 mg Cholesterol; 0 g Carbohydrate; 0 g Fibre; 24 g Protein; 57 mg Sodium

CHOICES: 3 Meat & Alternatives

Pictured on page 53.

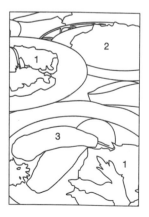

1. Fish Parcels, page 21
2. Shrimp and Asparagus Stir-Fry, page 33
3. Parmesan-Crumbed Fish, page 25

Props courtesy of: Pier 1 Imports

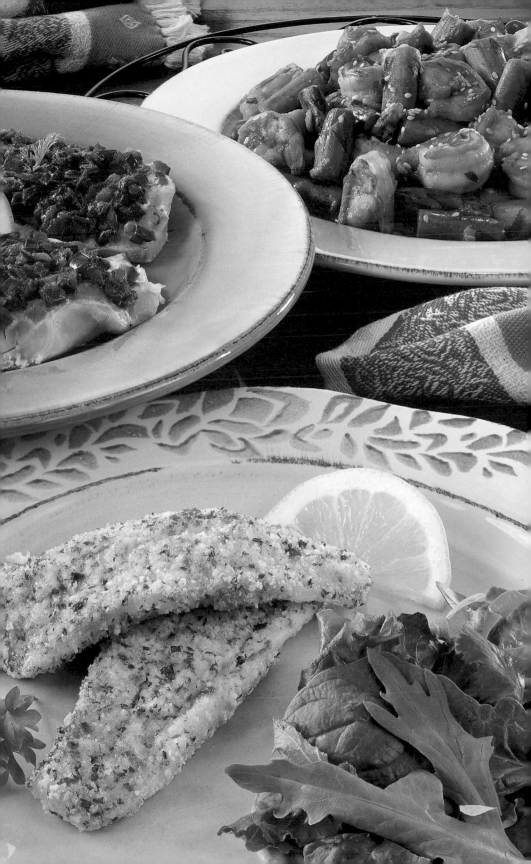

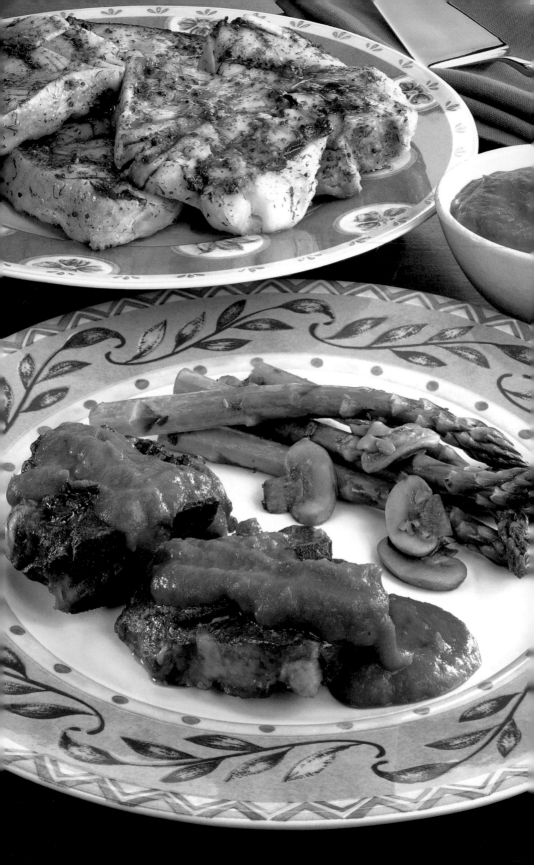

Succulent Lamb Chops

Juicy lamb chops flavoured with lime and chili. Adjust the chili sauce to suit your taste.

Lime juice	1/4 cup	60 mL
Sweet chili sauce	3 tbsp.	50 mL
Oyster sauce	1 tbsp.	15 mL
Finely grated lime zest	1 tsp.	5 mL
Garlic clove, minced	1	1
(or 1/4 tsp., 1 mL, powder)		
Rack of lamb (with 8 ribs), trimmed of fat and cut into chops	1	1

Combine first 5 ingredients in medium bowl.

Add lamb chops. Turn until coated. Cover. Marinate in refrigerator for at least 8 hours or overnight. Drain and discard marinade. Preheat electric grill for 5 minutes or gas barbecue to medium-high. Cook chops on greased grill for about 5 minutes per side until tender and desired doneness. Serves 4.

1 serving: 205 Calories; 15.5 g Total Fat (6.4 g Mono, 1.3 g Poly, 6.6 g Sat); 57 mg Cholesterol; 2 g Carbohydrate; trace Fibre; 13 g Protein; 97 mg Sodium

CHOICES: 2 Meat & Alternatives

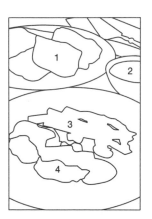

1. Mustard Dill Halibut, page 66
2. Spicy Roasted Pepper Sauce, page 112
3. Asparagus And Mushrooms, page 109
4. Peppered Lamb, page 73, with Spicy Roasted Pepper Sauce, page 113

Props courtesy of: Danesco Inc.

Pepper Pork Skewers

Bright and colourful skewers with tender pork. Serve with Crunchy Rice Salad, page 97.

Lime juice	3 tbsp.	50 mL
Apricot jam	2 tbsp.	30 mL
Dijon mustard (with whole seeds)	2 tbsp.	30 mL
Garlic clove, minced (or 1/4 tsp., 1 mL, powder)	1	1
Low-sodium soy sauce	1 tbsp.	15 mL
Pork tenderloin, trimmed of fat and cut into 1 inch (2.5 cm) cubes	1 lb.	454 g
Small red pepper, cut into 1 inch (2.5 cm) pieces	1	1
Small yellow pepper, cut into 1 inch (2.5 cm) pieces	1	1
Bamboo skewers (8 inch, 20 cm, length), soaked in water for 10 minutes	8	8
Lemon pepper	1 tsp.	5 mL

Combine first 5 ingredients in large bowl.

Add pork. Toss until coated. Cover. Marinate in refrigerator for at least 3 hours. Drain and discard marinade.

Thread pork and red and yellow peppers alternately onto skewers.

Sprinkle with lemon pepper. Preheat electric grill for 5 minutes or gas barbecue to medium-high. Cook skewers on greased grill for 15 to 20 minutes, turning occasionally, until pork is tender. Makes 8 skewers. Serves 4.

1 serving: 154 Calories; 4.1 g Total Fat (1.8 g Mono, 0.5 g Poly, 1.4 g Sat); 74 mg Cholesterol; 4 g Carbohydrate; 1 g Fibre; 24 g Protein; 127 mg Sodium

CHOICES: 3 Meat & Alternatives

Pictured on page 89.

Warm Pork Salad

Lightly dressed spinach with the sweetness of dates.

Sesame oil	1 tsp.	5 mL
Pork tenderloin, trimmed of fat and cut into 1/4 inch (6 mm) strips	1 lb.	454 g
Fresh spinach leaves (cut or torn if large), lightly packed	6 cups	1.5 L
Coarsely chopped pitted dates	1/2 cup	125 mL
Medium Roma (plum) tomatoes, quartered lengthwise	3	3
MUSTARD MAYONNAISE DRESSING		
Orange juice	1/4 cup	60 mL
Low-fat mayonnaise	1/4 cup	60 mL
Dijon mustard (with whole seeds)	1 tbsp.	15 mL
Salt	1/4 tsp.	1 mL
Sesame seeds, toasted (see Tip, page 97)	1 tbsp.	15 mL

Heat wok or large frying pan on medium-high until very hot. Add sesame oil. Add pork. Stir-fry for about 5 minutes until tender and lightly browned. Transfer to large bowl.

Add next 3 ingredients. Toss gently.

Mustard Mayonnaise Dressing: Combine first 4 ingredients in jar with tight-fitting lid. Shake well. Makes about 1/2 cup (125 mL) mayonnaise. Drizzle over salad. Toss.

Sprinkle with sesame seeds. Makes about 9 1/2 cups (2.4 L). Serves 6.

1 serving: 183 Calories; 5.8 g Total Fat (1.2 g Mono, 0.4 g Poly, 1.4 g Sat); 49 mg Cholesterol; 16 g Carbohydrate; 2 g Fibre; 18 g Protein; 301 mg Sodium

CHOICES: 2 Meat & Alternatives; 1/2 Fruits; 1/2 Fats

Pictured on page 53.

Kid-Friendly Idea: Substitute same amount of chopped romaine lettuce for the spinach. Omit dates.

1 serving: 145 Calories; 5.8 g Total Fat (1.2 g Mono, 0.4 g Poly, 1.4 g Sat); 49 mg Cholesterol; 6 g Carbohydrate; 2 g Fibre; 17 g Protein; 281 mg Sodium

CHOICES: 2 Meat & Alternatives; 1/2 Fats

Artichoke and Ham Pie

An attractive meat pie with red peppers and artichokes peeking through. Great for brunch, lunch or a light dinner. Can be prepared the day before and chilled for up to 24 hours before baking.

Whole-wheat bread slices, cut into 1 inch (2.5 cm) pieces	4	4
Chopped low-fat deli ham	1 cup	250 mL
Can of artichoke hearts, drained, chopped	14 oz.	398 mL
Diced roasted red peppers	1/4 cup	60 mL
Finely grated fresh Parmesan cheese	1/3 cup	75 mL
Can of skim evaporated milk	13 1/2 oz.	385 mL
Non-fat creamed cottage cheese	1/2 cup	125 mL
Large eggs	4	4
Egg whites (large)	2	2
All-purpose flour	1 tbsp.	15 mL
Garlic cloves, halved (or 3/4 tsp., 4 mL, powder)	3	3
Ground nutmeg	1/8 tsp.	0.5 mL
Paprika	1/4 tsp.	1 mL
Pepper	1/4 tsp.	1 mL

Spray 10 inch (25 cm) pie plate or 9 inch (23 cm) deep-dish pie plate with cooking spray. Layer first 5 ingredients in plate in order given.

Process next 7 ingredients in blender or food processor until almost smooth. Pour over layers. Cover. Chill for at least 6 hours.

Sprinkle with paprika and pepper. Bake, uncovered, in 375°F (190°C) oven for 55 to 60 minutes until edge is golden and pie is evenly puffed across centre. Let stand for 10 minutes. Cuts into 6 wedges.

1 wedge: 278 Calories; 9.1 g Total Fat (0.5 g Mono, 0.2 g Poly, 3.6 g Sat); 159 mg Cholesterol; 26 g Carbohydrate; 1 g Fibre; 22 g Protein; 978 mg Sodium

CHOICES: 1/2 Grains & Starches; 1 Vegetables; 1 1/2 Meat & Alternatives

Stuffed Zucchini

These "boats" are always so appealing in the late summer when zucchini are in abundance. Mushrooms and cheese complement the zucchini.

Large zucchini (with peel)	2	2
Olive oil	1 tsp.	5 mL
Olive oil	2 tsp.	10 mL
Chopped fresh brown mushrooms	2 cups	500 mL
Garlic clove, minced	1	1
(or 1/4 tsp., 1 mL, powder)		
Lemon pepper	1/2 tsp.	2 mL
Grated part-skim mozzarella cheese	3/4 cup	175 mL
Finely chopped fresh oregano	1 tbsp.	15 mL
(or 3/4 tsp., 4 mL, dried)		
Crumbled light feta cheese	1/4 cup	60 mL

Cut off both ends of zucchini. Cut in half lengthwise. Remove flesh using small spoon, leaving 1/4 inch (6 mm) thick shell. Reserve flesh in small bowl. Brush cut sides of zucchini lightly with first amount of olive oil. Place, cut side up, in ungreased shallow baking pan. Bake in 400°F (205°C) oven for about 15 minutes until softened.

Heat second amount of olive oil in large non-stick frying pan on medium. Add reserved zucchini and next 3 ingredients. Stir. Cook for about 10 minutes, stirring often, until liquid is evaporated. Transfer to medium bowl. Cool for 10 minutes.

Add cheese and oregano. Makes about 1 cup (250 mL) stuffing. Spoon into zucchini shells.

Sprinkle feta cheese over stuffing. Bake, uncovered, in 400°F (205°C) oven for about 15 minutes until heated through. Makes 4 stuffed zucchini.

1 stuffed zucchini: 148 Calories; 9.7 g Total Fat (2.5 g Mono, 0.6 g Poly, 4.1 g Sat); 16 mg Cholesterol; 8.5 g Carbohydrate; 2 g Fibre; 11 g Protein; 338 mg Sodium

CHOICES: 1 Meat & Alternatives; 1 Vegetables; 1/2 Fats

Kid-Friendly Idea: Substitute same amount of grated light Monterey Jack cheese for the feta cheese.

1 stuffed zucchini: 161 Calories; 11.0 g Total Fat (2.5 g Mono, 0.6 g Poly, 4.7 g Sat); 20 mg Cholesterol; 8 g Carbohydrate; 2 g Fibre; 11 g Protein; 282 mg Sodium

CHOICES: 1 Vegetables; 1 Meat & Alternatives; 1/2 Fats

Vegetable Lasagna

Make this delicious dish the day before and pop it in the oven after work.
Serve with a tossed green salad and fresh tomatoes.

Boiling water	12 cups	3 L
Salt	2 tsp.	10 mL
Whole-wheat lasagna noodles	6	6
Olive oil	1 tbsp.	15 mL
Broccoli slaw	2 cups	500 mL
Diced zucchini (with peel)	2 cups	500 mL
Sliced fresh brown mushrooms	2 cups	500 mL
Coarsely grated carrot	3/4 cup	175 mL
Medium onion, chopped	1	1
Garlic cloves, minced	2	2
(or 1/2 tsp., 2 mL, powder)		
Can of stewed tomatoes (with juice), chopped	14 oz.	398 mL
Tomato paste (see Tip, page 43)	2 tbsp.	30 mL
Chopped fresh basil	3 tbsp.	50 mL
(or 2 1/4 tsp., 11 mL, dried)		
Chopped fresh parsley	3 tbsp.	50 mL
(or 2 1/4 tsp., 11 mL, flakes)		
Pepper	1/2 tsp.	2 mL
Non-fat cottage cheese	2 cups	500 mL
Large eggs	2	2
Fresh spinach leaves, lightly packed	2 cups	500 mL
Finely grated fresh Parmesan cheese	1/3 cup	75 mL
Skim evaporated milk	2/3 cup	150 mL
Garlic and herb no-salt seasoning	1 tsp.	5 mL
Grated part-skim mozzarella cheese	1 cup	250 mL

Combine boiling water and salt in large pot or Dutch oven. Add noodles. Cook, uncovered, for 10 minutes, stirring often. Noodles will still be firm. Drain. Rinse with cold water. Set aside.

(continued on next page)

Heat wok or large frying pan on medium-high until very hot. Add olive oil. Add next 6 ingredients. Stir-fry for 5 minutes. Cook, uncovered, for 4 to 5 minutes, stirring occasionally, until vegetables are soft and liquid is evaporated.

Add next 5 ingredients. Stir. Remove from heat. Spread 1 cup (250 mL) evenly in greased 9 x 13 inch (23 x 33 cm) dish. Arrange 3 noodles over top. Spread half of remaining sauce over top.

Put next 6 ingredients into blender. Pulse with on/off motion, scraping down sides as necessary, until smooth. Spread about 1 3/4 cups (425 mL) evenly over tomato mixture. Layer remaining noodles, remaining tomato mixture and cottage cheese mixture, in order given, over top.

Sprinkle with mozzarella cheese. Cover tightly with greased foil. Bake in 325°F (160°C) oven for 45 minutes. Remove foil. Bake at 375°F (190°C) for about 15 minutes until edges are golden. Let stand on wire rack for 15 minutes before cutting. Serves 6.

1 serving: 333 Calories; 10.5 g Total Fat (1.7 g Mono, 0.5 g Poly, 4.6 g Sat); 92 mg Cholesterol; 37 g Carbohydrate; 4 g Fibre; 26 g Protein; 783 mg Sodium

CHOICES: 1 Grains & Starches; 2 Vegetables; 2 Meat & Alternatives; 1/2 Fats

Pictured on page 54.

Kid-Friendly Idea: Finely chop all the vegetables so there aren't any large pieces. Reduce amount of basil.

 To store tomato paste when a recipe doesn't call for a whole can, freeze unopened can for 30 minutes. Open both ends and push contents through, slicing off only what you need. Freeze remaining tomato paste in resealable freezer bag for future use.

Bows and Fresh Vegetables

A creamy garlic sauce coats colourful vegetables and bow pasta. Have your vegetables cut before cooking the pasta. The flavours are enhanced by a pinch of salt, if your diet permits.

Boiling water	12 cups	3 L
Salt	1 tbsp.	15 mL
Medium bow pasta	3 cups	750 mL
Broccoli florets	1 cup	250 mL
Chopped fresh asparagus	1 cup	250 mL
Small red pepper, diced	1	1
Fresh snow peas	1 cup	250 mL
Skim milk	1 1/2 cups	375 mL
All-purpose flour	2 tbsp.	30 mL
Garlic powder	1/4 tsp.	1 mL
Grated part-skim mozzarella cheese	1/2 cup	125 mL
Chopped fresh parsley	1 tbsp.	15 mL
(or 3/4 tsp., 4 mL, flakes)		
Finely grated fresh Parmesan cheese	1 tbsp.	15 mL
Pepper	1/4 tsp.	1 mL

Combine boiling water and salt in large pot or Dutch oven. Add pasta. Cook, uncovered, for 6 minutes, stirring occasionally. Do not drain.

Add broccoli and asparagus. Bring to a boil. Cook, uncovered, for 2 minutes.

Add red pepper and snow peas. Bring to a boil. Cook, uncovered, for about 3 minutes until pasta is tender but firm. Drain. Return to pot. Cover to keep warm.

Stir milk into flour in medium saucepan until smooth. Add garlic powder. Heat and stir on medium for about 10 minutes until boiling and thickened.

Add cheese. Stir until melted. Pour over pasta mixture. Toss. Transfer to warm serving bowl.

Sprinkle with remaining 3 ingredients just before serving. Makes about 7 cups (1.75 L). Serves 4.

(continued on next page)

1 serving: 331 Calories; 4.8 g Total Fat (trace Mono, 0.1 g Poly, 2.2 g Sat); 11 mg Cholesterol; 55 g Carbohydrate; 4 g Fibre; 17 g Protein; 183 mg Sodium

CHOICES: 3 Grains & Starches; 1/2 Meat & Alternatives

Kid-Friendly Idea: Use kid-friendly vegetables like carrots and sugar snap peas instead of the broccoli, asparagus, red pepper and/or snow peas. Remember to add firmer vegetables after pasta has cooked for 6 minutes and softer vegetables nearer the end of cooking time.

1 serving: 361 Calories; 4.7 g Total Fat (trace Mono, 0.1 g Poly, 2.2 g Sat); 11 mg Cholesterol; 62 g Carbohydrate; 5 g Fibre; 17 g Protein; 227 mg Sodium

CHOICES: 3 Grains & Starches; 1 1/2 Vegetables; 1/2 Meat & Alternatives

Roasted Red Pepper Pizza

A delicious, easy-to-prepare pizza with a flavourful topping.

Prebaked pizza crust (12 inch, 30 cm, diameter)	1	1
Pizza sauce	1/3 cup	75 mL
Chopped roasted red peppers	1 cup	250 mL
Fresh spinach leaves, lightly packed	1 cup	250 mL
Thinly sliced red onion	1 cup	250 mL
Chopped fresh basil (or 1 1/2 tsp., 7 mL, dried)	2 tbsp.	30 mL
Crumbled light feta cheese	1/3 cup	75 mL
Finely grated fresh Parmesan cheese	3 tbsp.	50 mL

Place pizza crust on ungreased 12 inch (30 cm) pizza pan or baking sheet. Spread pizza sauce evenly over crust.

Layer remaining 6 ingredients, in order given, over sauce. Bake on lowest rack in 475°F (240°C) oven for about 20 minutes until crust is browned. Cuts into 8 wedges.

1 wedge: 113 Calories; 2.5 g Total Fat (0 g Mono, trace Poly, 1.1 g Sat); 6 mg Cholesterol; 16 g Carbohydrate; 1 g Fibre; 5 g Protein; 506 mg Sodium

CHOICES: 1 Vegetables; 1/2 Grains & Starches

Pictured on page 54.

Spinach and Cheese Roll

Lovely golden, flaky pastry and subtle, tangy feta flavour. Serve with a crisp lettuce and tomato salad.

Olive oil	2 tsp.	10 mL
Finely chopped onion	1 cup	250 mL
Garlic cloves, minced	4	4
(or 1 tsp., 5 mL, powder)		
Boxes of frozen chopped spinach	2	2
(10 oz., 300 g, each), thawed and		
squeezed dry, chopped finer		
Lemon pepper	1/2 tsp.	2 mL
Ground nutmeg	1/4 tsp.	1 mL
Part-skim ricotta cheese, drained	1/2 cup	125 mL
Crumbled light feta cheese	1/2 cup	125 mL
Chopped fresh parsley	3 tbsp.	50 mL
(or 2 1/4 tsp., 11 mL, flakes)		
Phyllo pastry sheets, thawed	6	6
according to package directions		
ROASTED PEPPER SAUCE		
Jar of roasted red peppers, drained and	13 oz.	370 mL
blotted dry		
Balsamic vinegar	1 tbsp.	15 mL
Brown sugar, packed	1 tsp.	5 mL
Lemon pepper	1/4 tsp.	1 mL

Heat olive oil in large non-stick frying pan on medium. Add onion and garlic. Cook for about 5 minutes, stirring often, until onion is softened.

Add spinach to onion mixture. Add lemon pepper and nutmeg. Stir. Cook for 1 to 2 minutes, stirring often, until heated through and liquid is evaporated. Transfer to medium bowl. Cool to room temperature.

Add next 3 ingredients. Stir well.

(continued on next page)

Lay tea towel, short end closest to you, on work surface. Place 1 phyllo sheet, short end closest to you, on tea towel. Cover remaining sheets with damp tea towel to prevent drying out. Lightly spray first sheet with cooking spray. Place second sheet on top of first. Working quickly, lightly spray with cooking spray. Repeat with remaining sheets. Mound spinach filling evenly along short end of pastry closest to you, 6 inches (15 cm) from bottom edge, leaving about 1 inch (2.5 cm) on either side. Fold bottom edge of sheets up and over filling. Roll firmly to enclose filling, using tea towel as a guide. Pack any loose filling back into roll. Do not tuck in sides. Place, seam-side down, on greased baking sheet with sides. Spray with cooking spray. Bake in 400°F (205°C) oven for 15 to 20 minutes until golden brown. Cut into twelve 1 inch (2.5 cm) slices.

Roasted Pepper Sauce: Process all 4 ingredients in blender until smooth. Pour into medium saucepan. Heat on medium, stirring occasionally, until boiling. Reduce heat to medium-low. Simmer, uncovered, for 5 minutes. Makes 3/4 cup (175 mL) sauce. Spoon sauce over slices. Serves 6.

1 serving: 251 Calories; 7.2 g Total Fat (1.7 g Mono, 0.4 g Poly, 3.3 g Sat); 18 mg Cholesterol; 31 g Carbohydrate; 3 g Fibre; 12 g Protein; 1108 mg Sodium

CHOICES: 3 Vegetables; 1 Meat & Alternatives

Kid-Friendly Idea: Substitute about 1 1/2 cups (375 mL) of finely chopped carrot for the spinach. Replace feta cheese with light sharp Cheddar cheese.

1 serving: 255 Calories; 7.8 g Total Fat (1.7 g Mono, 0.5 g Poly, 3.8 g Sat); 21 mg Cholesterol; 30 g Carbohydrate; 2 g Fibre; 11 g Protein; 927 mg Sodium

CHOICES: 3 Vegetables; 1 Meat & Alternatives

Paré Pointer

Sammy thought that the highest form of animal life was a giraffe.

Chicken Cacciatore

Tender chicken and fresh vegetables rest in a rich, red tomato sauce. Serve the excess sauce over pasta. Delicious!

All-purpose flour	2 tbsp.	30 mL
Paprika	1/2 tsp.	2 mL
Salt	1/4 tsp.	1 mL
Pepper	1/4 tsp.	1 mL
Boneless, skinless chicken thighs, halved	1 lb.	454 g
Chopped onion	3/4 cup	175 mL
Chopped red pepper	1/2 cup	125 mL
Chopped green pepper	1/2 cup	125 mL
Garlic cloves, minced	2	2
(or 1/2 tsp., 2 mL, powder)		
Can of diced tomatoes (with juice)	28 oz.	796 mL
Sliced fresh white mushrooms	2 cups	500 mL
Tomato paste (see Tip, page 43)	1/4 cup	60 mL
Balsamic vinegar	1 tbsp.	15 mL
Granulated sugar	1/2 tsp.	2 mL

Combine first 4 ingredients in large plastic bag.

Add chicken. Seal. Toss until coated. Shake excess flour mixture from chicken. Discard any remaining flour. Transfer to 3 quart (3 L) casserole. Cover. Microwave on high (100%) for 3 minutes. Turn chicken. Cover. Microwave on high (100%) for 2 to 3 minutes until no longer pink inside. Transfer chicken to plate. Cover to keep warm.

Combine next 4 ingredients in same casserole. Cover. Microwave on high (100%) for 5 to 7 minutes until vegetables are tender. Stir.

Add chicken and remaining 5 ingredients. Stir. Cover. Microwave on high (100%) for 5 minutes. Stir. Cover. Microwave on high (100%) for 10 to 12 minutes until chicken is tender. Serves 4.

1 serving: 261 Calories; 8.7 g Total Fat (3.3 g Mono, 2.0 g Poly, 2.4 g Sat); 74 mg Cholesterol; 22 g Carbohydrate; 2 g Fibre; 24 g Protein; 774 mg Sodium

CHOICES: 3 Vegetables; 3 Meat & Alternatives

Pictured on page 71.

Kid-Friendly Idea: Substitute same amount of white vinegar for the balsamic.

Turkey in Curry Sauce

A rich, yellow curry sauce coats chunks of turkey and soft mango.

Chopped onion	1 cup	250 mL
Flake coconut	2 tbsp.	30 mL
Canola oil	2 tsp.	10 mL
Curry powder	2 tsp.	10 mL
Chili powder	1/4 tsp.	1 mL
Ground cinnamon	1/4 tsp.	1 mL
All-purpose flour	2 tsp.	10 mL
2% evaporated milk	1 cup	250 mL
Boneless, skinless turkey breast halves, diced	1 lb.	454 g
Can of sliced mango in light syrup, drained and diced	14 oz.	398 mL
Hot cooked jasmine rice (about 2 cups, 500 mL, uncooked)	4 cups	1 L

Combine first 6 ingredients in ungreased 1 1/2 quart (1.5 L) casserole. Cover. Microwave on high (100%) for 3 minutes, stirring twice.

Sprinkle flour over onion mixture. Stir. Cover. Microwave on high (100%) for about 1 minute until onion is softened.

Add evaporated milk. Stir. Cover. Microwave on high (100%) for 1 to 2 minutes until boiling and slightly thickened.

Add turkey. Stir until coated. Cover. Microwave on high (100%) for 4 minutes, stirring once at halftime.

Add mango. Stir. Cover. Microwave on medium (50%) for 3 minutes, stirring once at halftime. Let stand for 2 minutes. Makes about 3 3/4 cups (925 mL).

Spoon over rice. Serves 4.

1 serving: 470 Calories; 6.0 g Total Fat (1.8 g Mono, 0.8 g Poly, 1.6 g Sat); 50 mg Cholesterol; 71 g Carbohydrate; 3 g Fibre; 37 g Protein; 147 mg Sodium

CHOICES: 2 Grains & Starches; 1 1/2 Fruits; 1/2 Milk & Alternatives; 1/2 Fats

 tip To ensure even cooking in a microwave, rotate dish half a turn halfway through cooking time.

Asian Rice Bowl

A wonderful, fresh-tasting dish with a variety of crunchy vegetables and a lingering heat.

Brown converted rice	1 cup	250 mL
Hot water	2 cups	500 mL
Finely chopped onion	1/2 cup	125 mL
Sweet chili sauce	1 tbsp.	15 mL
Garlic cloves, minced	2	2
(or 1/2 tsp., 2 mL, powder)		
Dried crushed chilies	1/4 tsp.	1 mL
Lean ground chicken	8 oz.	225 g
Green onions, sliced	4	4
Dry sherry	1 tbsp.	15 mL
Low-sodium soy sauce	2 tbsp.	30 mL
Rice vinegar	4 tsp.	20 mL
Cornstarch	2 tsp.	10 mL
Cooked salad shrimp	4 oz.	113 g
Fresh bean sprouts	2 cups	500 mL
Green onion, sliced	1	1
Julienned English cucumber (with peel)	1/4 cup	60 mL

Combine rice and hot water in ungreased 2 quart (2 L) casserole. Cover. Microwave on high (100%) for 12 minutes. Let stand for 10 minutes.

Combine next 4 ingredients in ungreased 1 quart (1 L) casserole. Cover. Microwave on high (100%) for 2 minutes. Stir.

Add next 3 ingredients. Stir. Cover. Microwave on high (100%) for 4 minutes, stirring once at halftime.

Stir next 3 ingredients in small cup until smooth. Add to chicken mixture. Stir. Cover. Microwave on high (100%) for about 1 minute until boiling and slightly thickened. Add to rice. Stir. Add shrimp and bean sprouts. Stir. Cover. Microwave on high (100%) for about 2 minutes until heated through. Spoon into 4 serving bowls.

Top with second amount of green onion and cucumber. Serves 4.

(continued on next page)

Microwave

1 serving: 353 Calories; 6.6 g Total Fat (0.6 g Mono, 0.8 g Poly, 1.7 g Sat); 81 mg Cholesterol; 52 g Carbohydrate; 4 g Fibre; 23 g Protein; 389 mg Sodium

CHOICES: 2 Grains & Starches; 2 Vegetables; 2 Meat & Alternatives

Kid-Friendly Idea: Substitute long grain white rice for the brown converted rice. Omit chili sauce, dried crushed chilies and green onions. Substitute one 4 oz. (113 g) chicken breast half, diced, for the shrimp.

1 serving: 356 Calories; 5.5 g Total Fat (0.3 g Mono, 0.3 g Poly, 1.5 g Sat); 54 mg Cholesterol; 53 g Carbohydrate; 3 g Fibre; 24 g Protein; 325 mg Sodium

CHOICES: 2 1/2 Grains & Starches; 2 Vegetables; 2 Meat & Alternatives

---

Roasted Lamb Rack

Succulent lamb chops covered with a glossy honey garlic sauce. These are quick and so easy to prepare.

Liquid honey	2 tbsp.	30 mL
Low-sodium soy sauce	1 tbsp.	15 mL
Dried rosemary, crushed	1 tsp.	5 mL
Garlic powder	1/2 tsp.	2 mL
Pepper	1/4 tsp.	1 ml
Rack of lamb (with 8 ribs), trimmed of fat	13 oz.	370 g

Combine first 5 ingredients in small bowl.

Place lamb rack, meat-side up, in shallow microwave-safe dish. Brush with honey mixture. Turn over. Microwave, uncovered, on high (100%) for 5 minutes. Turn over. Microwave, uncovered, on high (100%) for 2 to 4 minutes until meat thermometer registers 140°F to 160°F (60°C to 70°C) when inserted into thickest part of meat or until desired doneness. Cover. Let stand for 5 minutes. Cut rack into chops. Makes 8 chops. Serves 4.

1 serving: 198 Calories; 12.7 g Total Fat (5.2 g Mono, 1.0 g Poly, 5.4 g Sat); 46 mg Cholesterol; 9 g Carbohydrate; trace Fibre; 11 g Protein; 170 mg Sodium

CHOICES: 1/2 Other Choices; 1 1/2 Meat & Alternatives

Chicken Stroganoff

A savoury variation which uses cream cheese instead of sour cream.

Sliced fresh white mushrooms	2 cups	500 mL
Thinly sliced onion	1 cup	250 mL
Canola oil	2 tsp.	10 mL
Paprika	1/2 tsp.	2 mL
Garlic clove, minced	1	1
(or 1/4 tsp., 1 mL, powder)		
Boneless, skinless chicken thighs, cut into thin strips	1 lb.	454 g
Tomato paste (see Tip, page 43)	1/4 cup	60 mL
Salt	1/4 tsp.	1 mL
Pepper	1/4 tsp.	1 mL
Chopped light cream cheese, softened	1/4 cup	60 mL
Low-sodium prepared chicken broth	1/4 cup	60 mL
Cornstarch	2 tsp.	10 mL

Combine first 5 ingredients in ungreased 2 quart (2 L) casserole. Cover. Microwave on high (100%) for 8 minutes, stirring once at halftime.

Add next 4 ingredients. Stir. Cover. Microwave on high (100%) for about 8 minutes, stirring once at halftime, until chicken is tender. Stir.

Add cream cheese. Stir.

Stir broth into cornstarch in small bowl until smooth. Add to chicken mixture. Stir. Cover. Microwave on high (100%) for 1 minute. Stir. Microwave on high (100%) for about 1 minute until hot and cheese is melted. Makes about 3 cups (750 mL). Serves 4.

1 serving: 262 Calories; 13.5 g Total Fat (4.6 g Mono, 2.6 g Poly, 4.3 g Sat); 82 mg Cholesterol; 10 g Carbohydrate; 2 g Fibre; 23 g Protein; 343 mg Sodium

CHOICES: 1 Vegetables; 3 Meat & Alternatives; 1/2 Fats

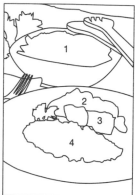

1. Warm Pork Salad, page 39
2. Apple Cranberry Chutney, page 116
3. Maple Balsamic Tenderloin, page 34
4. Spinach Mushroom Rice, page 93

Props courtesy of: Cherison Enterprises Inc.

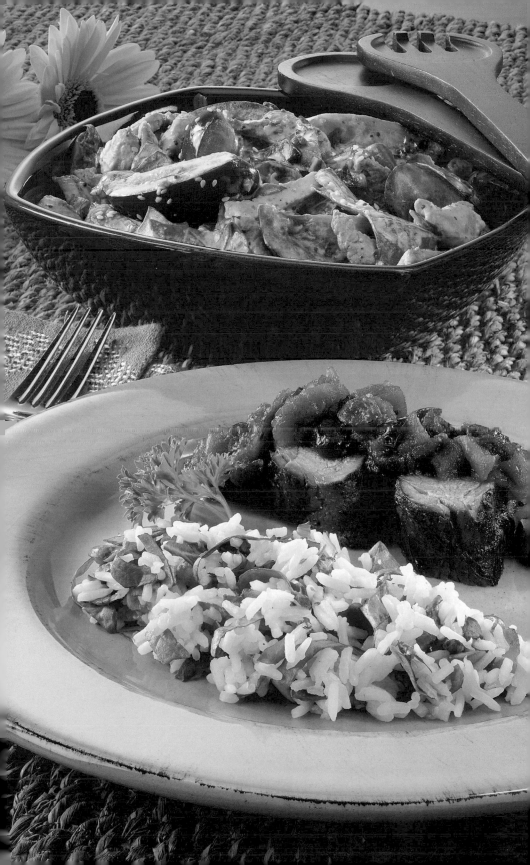

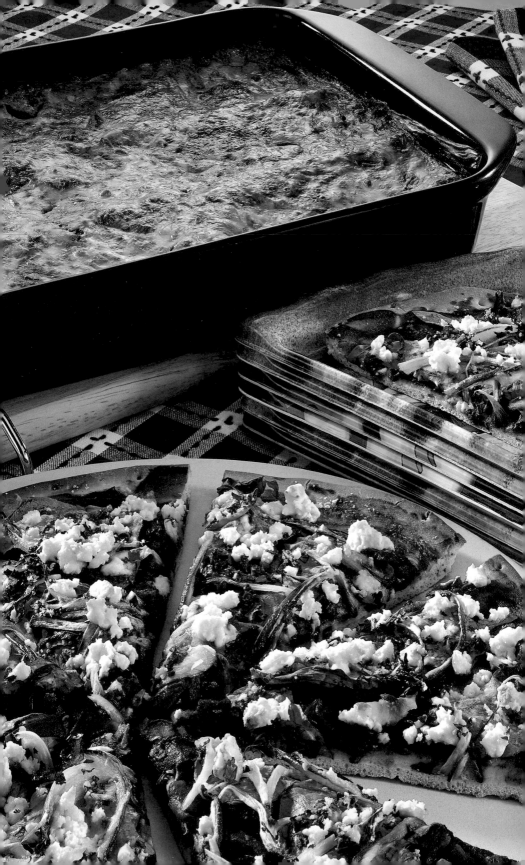

Mustard Honey Salmon

Moist, perfectly cooked salmon with a delicious honey mustard glaze. Serve with a crisp green salad or Easy Couscous, page 92.

Dijon mustard	2 tbsp.	30 mL
Chopped fresh parsley	2 tbsp.	30 mL
(or 1 1/2 tsp., 7 mL, flakes)		
Liquid honey	2 tbsp.	30 mL
Garlic salt	1/2 tsp.	2 mL
Salmon fillets, skin and any small bones removed (about 3/4 inch, 2 cm, thick), 5 oz. (140 g) each	4	4

Combine first 4 ingredients in small bowl.

Place salmon in shallow microwave-safe dish. Brush mustard mixture over salmon. Cover. Microwave on high (100%) for 4 to 5 minutes until salmon flakes easily when tested with fork. Let stand for 2 minutes. Serves 4.

1 serving: 288 Calories; 14.8 g Total Fat (6.2 g Mono, 4.0 g Poly, 4.4 g Sat); 71 mg Cholesterol; 9 g Carbohydrate; trace Fibre; 28 g Protein; 285 mg Sodium

CHOICES: 1/2 Other Choices; 4 Meat & Alternatives

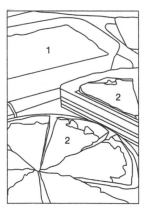

1. Vegetable Lasagna, page 42
2. Roasted Red Pepper Pizza, page 45

Pasta and Cheese Supper

A warm, cheesy sauce coats perfectly cooked whole-wheat pasta. Serve with a fresh garden salad.

Boiling water	10 cups	2.5 L
Salt	2 tsp.	10 mL
Whole-wheat rotini pasta	2 2/3 cups	650 mL
Olive oil	1 tbsp.	15 mL
Finely chopped onion	2/3 cup	150 mL
All-purpose flour	1/4 cup	60 mL
Dry mustard	1/2 tsp.	2 mL
Salt	1/4 tsp.	1 mL
Pepper	1/4 tsp.	1 mL
Milk	2 cups	500 mL
Non-fat cottage cheese, mashed (or processed) until almost smooth	1 cup	250 mL
Grated light sharp Cheddar cheese	1 cup	250 mL
Grated part-skim mozzarella cheese	1 cup	250 mL

Combine boiling water and salt in large pot or Dutch oven. Add pasta. Cook, uncovered, for 10 to 12 minutes, stirring occasionally, until tender but firm. Drain. Rinse with cold water. Drain well. Return to pot to keep warm.

Combine olive oil and onion in ungreased 3 quart (3 L) casserole. Cover. Microwave on high (100%) for about 4 minutes, stirring once at halftime, until onion is softened.

Add next 4 ingredients. Stir. Gradually whisk in milk. Cover. Microwave on medium (50%) for 4 minutes. Stir with whisk. Cover. Microwave on medium (50%) for 8 to 10 minutes, stirring twice, until boiling and thickened.

Add remaining 3 ingredients. Stir well. Add pasta. Toss. Spread evenly. Cover. Microwave on medium (50%) for 10 minutes. Let stand for 2 minutes before serving. Makes 6 cups (1.5 L). Serves 4.

1 serving: 489 Calories; 16.2 g Total Fat (3.0 g Mono, 0.5 g Poly, 7.9 g Sat); 40 mg Cholesterol; 56 g Carbohydrate; 3 g Fibre; 34 g Protein; 776 mg Sodium

CHOICES: 2 1/2 Grains & Starches; 1/2 Milk & Alternatives; 3 Meat & Alternatives; 1/2 Fats

Beef and Tomato Stew

A vibrant, saucy stew with a wonderful variety of fresh flavours and textures.
A quick, easy dish that goes well with a salad or hot vegetables.

Thinly sliced onion	1 1/2 cups	375 mL
Garlic cloves, minced	2	2
(or 1/2 tsp., 2 mL, powder)		
Olive oil	2 tsp.	10 mL
Beef sirloin tip steak, cut into 2 inch (5 cm) strips	3/4 lb.	340 g
Water	1/2 cup	125 mL
All-purpose flour	1 1/2 tbsp.	25 mL
Can of stewed tomatoes (with juice), broken up	14 oz.	398 mL
Paprika (Hungarian is best)	2 tsp.	10 mL
Low-sodium beef bouillon powder	1 tsp.	5 mL
Granulated sugar	1 tsp.	5 mL
Dried marjoram	1/2 tsp.	2 mL
Worcestershire sauce	1/2 tsp.	2 mL
Pepper	1/4 tsp.	1 mL
Light sour cream	2 tbsp.	30 mL
Balsamic vinegar	1 1/2 tsp.	7 mL

Combine first 3 ingredients in ungreased 2 quart (2 L) casserole. Cover. Microwave on high (100%) for about 4 minutes, stirring once at halftime, until onion is softened.

Add beef. Stir. Cover. Microwave on high (100%) for 3 minutes.

Stir water into flour in medium bowl until smooth. Add next 7 ingredients. Stir. Add to beef mixture. Stir. Cover. Microwave on medium (50%) for 10 to 12 minutes, stirring once at halftime, until sauce is boiling and thickened.

Add sour cream and vinegar. Stir. Makes 4 cups (1 L). Serves 4.

1 serving: 277 Calories; 12.5 g Total Fat (6.4 g Mono, 0.7 g Poly, 4.2 g Sat); 74 mg Cholesterol; 17 g Carbohydrate; 1 g Fibre; 24 g Protein; 402 mg Sodium

CHOICES: 2 Vegetables; 3 Meats & Alternatives; 1/2 Fats

Kid-Friendly Idea: Substitute same amount of white vinegar for the balsamic.

Apricot Beef Casserole

A richly flavoured gravy coats tender, moist strips of beef. Perfect served with couscous, rice or noodles.

Canola oil	2 tsp.	10 mL
Thinly sliced onion	1 cup	250 mL
All-purpose flour	1 tbsp.	15 mL
Curry powder	2 tsp.	10 mL
Ground cinnamon	1/4 tsp.	1 mL
Pepper	1/4 tsp.	1 mL
Beef sirloin tip steak, cut into thin strips	1 lb.	454 g
Liquid gravy browner	1/2 tsp.	2 mL
Apricot nectar	3/4 cup	175 mL
Chopped dried apricot	1/2 cup	125 mL
Worcestershire sauce	1 tsp.	5 mL
Chopped fresh parsley (or 1 1/2 tsp., 7 mL, flakes)	2 tbsp.	30 mL
Salt	1/4 tsp.	1 mL

Combine canola oil and onion in ungreased 2 quart (2 L) casserole. Cover. Microwave on high (100%) for about 5 minutes, stirring once at halftime, until onion is softened. Set aside.

Combine next 4 ingredients in large plastic bag.

Add beef. Seal. Toss until coated. Remove beef. Discard any remaining flour mixture. Add beef to onion. Stir. Drizzle with gravy browner. Stir. Cover. Microwave on high (100%) for 3 minutes. Stir.

Add next 3 ingredients. Stir. Cover. Microwave on medium (50%) for about 20 minutes, stirring once at halftime, until beef is tender.

Sprinkle with parsley and salt. Stir. Makes about 2 1/2 cups (625 mL). Serves 4.

1 serving: 304 Calories; 12.2 g Total Fat (6.2 g Mono, 1.2 g Poly, 3.8 g Sat); 74 mg Cholesterol; 24 g Carbohydrate; 2 g Fibre; 25 g Protein; 237 mg Sodium

CHOICES: 1 Fruits; 3 Meat & Alternatives; 1/2 Fats

Chicken Paprikash

Bite-size chunks of chicken rest in a tangy tomato sauce flavoured with paprika and green pepper. An easy-to-prepare dish that can be on the table in 30 minutes.

Boiling water	8 cups	2 L
Salt	2 tsp.	10 mL
Broad yolk-free egg noodles	5 cups	1.25 L
Chopped onion	1/2 cup	125 mL
Diced green pepper	1/2 cup	125 mL
Olive oil	2 tsp.	10 mL
Garlic cloves, minced (or 1/2 tsp., 2 mL, powder)	2	2
Boneless, skinless chicken breast halves, cut into 1 inch (2.5 cm) cubes	1 lb.	454 g
Can of tomato sauce	7 1/2 oz.	213 mL
Real bacon bits (or 2 slices, cooked crisp and crumbled)	2 tbsp.	30 mL
Paprika (Hungarian is best)	1 tbsp.	15 mL
Pepper	1/2 tsp.	2 mL
Light sour cream	1/2 cup	125 mL
All-purpose flour	2 tsp.	10 mL

Combine boiling water and salt in large pot or Dutch oven. Add noodles. Boil, uncovered, for 6 to 7 minutes, stirring occasionally, until tender but firm. Drain. Cover to keep warm.

Combine next 4 ingredients in ungreased 2 quart (2 L) casserole. Cover. Microwave on high (100%) for about 4 minutes, stirring once at halftime, until onion is softened.

Add next 5 ingredients. Stir. Cover. Microwave on high (100%) for about 7 minutes, stirring once at halftime, until chicken is no longer pink inside.

Stir sour cream into flour in small bowl until smooth. Add to chicken mixture. Stir. Cover. Microwave on medium (50%) for about 4 minutes until sauce is boiling and slightly thickened. Makes about 3 cups (750 mL). Toss with or spoon over noodles. Serves 4.

1 serving: 448 Calories; 8.1 g Total Fat (2.6 g Mono, 0.8 g Poly, 2.7 g Sat); 79 mg Cholesterol; 52 g Carbohydrate; 4 g Fibre; 38 g Protein; 510 mg Sodium

CHOICES: 2 1/2 Grains & Starches; 1 Vegetables; 4 Meats & Alternatives; 1 Fats

Peanut Butter Chicken

A saucy chicken dish. Serve with rice, noodles or couscous.

Olive oil	2 tsp.	10 mL
Medium onions, sliced	2	2
Garlic cloves, minced	2	2
(or 1/2 tsp., 2 mL, powder)		
Whole baby carrots	2 cups	500 mL
Bone-in chicken parts, skin removed	3 1/2 lbs.	1.6 kg
Can of tomato sauce	7 1/2 oz.	213 mL
Brown sugar, packed	1 tbsp.	15 mL
Curry powder	1 tsp.	5 mL
Peanut butter	1/2 cup	125 mL
Low-fat plain yogurt (not non-fat)	1/2 cup	125 mL
Olive oil	2 tsp.	10 mL
Medium zucchini (with peel), quartered lengthwise and cut crosswise into 3/4 inch (2 cm) pieces	2	2
Coarsely chopped unsalted peanuts	2 tbsp.	30 mL

Heat first amount of olive oil in large non-stick frying pan on medium. Add onion and garlic. Cook for about 10 minutes, stirring often, until onion is softened and starting to brown. Transfer to 3 1/2 quart (3.5 L) slow cooker.

Layer carrots and chicken over onion mixture. Do not stir.

Combine next 3 ingredients in small bowl. Spoon over chicken. Cover. Cook on Low for 7 to 8 hours or on High for 3 1/2 to 4 hours until chicken is no longer pink inside. Remove chicken to serving dish. Cover to keep warm.

Combine peanut butter and yogurt in small bowl. Add to slow cooker. Stir. Cover. Heat on Low for about 5 minutes until heated through.

Heat second amount of olive oil in large non-stick frying pan on medium-high. Add zucchini. Cook for about 5 minutes, stirring often, until slightly browned. Add to slow cooker. Stir. Pour sauce over chicken.

Sprinkle with peanuts. Makes 8 cups (2 L). Serves 8.

1 serving: 417 Calories; 18.3 g Total Fat (4.0 g Mono, 2.2 g Poly, 3.9 g Sat); 140 mg Cholesterol; 15 g Carbohydrate; 3 g Fibre; 49 g Protein; 405 mg Sodium

CHOICES: 1 Vegetables; 6 Meat & Alternatives; 2 Fats

Pictured on page 72.

Beef in Red Wine

A delicious and tender stew for very special occasions. Great served with mashed potatoes or noodles.

All-purpose flour	3 tbsp.	50 mL
Salt	1/4 tsp.	1 mL
Stewing beef, cut into 1 1/2 inch (3.8 cm) cubes	1 lb.	454 g
Canola oil	2 tsp.	10 mL
Thinly sliced onion	2 cups	500 mL
Thinly sliced carrot	1 cup	250 mL
Dry (or alcohol-free) red wine	1 cup	250 mL
Garlic cloves, minced (or 1/2 tsp., 2 mL, powder)	2	2
Sprig of fresh rosemary	1	1
Bay leaves	2	2
Pepper	1/4 tsp.	1 mL

Combine flour and salt in large plastic bag. Add beef. Shake until coated.

Heat canola oil in large frying pan on medium-high. Add beef. Cook for about 5 minutes, stirring occasionally, until browned. Transfer to 3 1/2 quart (3.5 L) slow cooker.

Add remaining 7 ingredients. Stir. Cover. Cook on Low for 6 to 8 hours or on High for 3 to 4 hours until beef is tender. Remove and discard rosemary sprig and bay leaves. Makes 3 cups (750 mL). Serves 4.

1 serving: 335 Calories; 16.8 g Total Fat (7.6 g Mono, 1.3 g Poly, 5.8 g Sat); 70 mg Cholesterol; 14 g Carbohydrate; 2 g Fibre; 21 g Protein; 215 mg Sodium

CHOICES: 1 Vegetables; 3 Meat & Alternatives

Kid-Friendly Idea: Although the alcohol in the wine will evaporate during cooking, you may prefer to substitute the same amount of low-sodium beef broth.

1 serving: 294 Calories; 17.2 g Total Fat (7.7 g Mono, 1.3 g Poly, 5.9 g Sat); 70 mg Cholesterol; 12 g Carbohydrate; 2 g Fibre; 22 g Protein; 231 mg sodium

CHOICES: 1/2 Starch; 1 Fruit & Vegetable; 3 1/2 Protein; 1/2 Fat & Oil

Slow Cooker Fajitas

Tender, spiced beef with both soft cooked and crisp, cold vegetables enclosed in a flour tortilla.

Beef sirloin tip steak, cut into 3 inch (7.5 cm) thin strips	1 1/2 lbs.	680 g
Thickly sliced fresh white mushrooms	2 cups	500 mL
Red medium pepper, cut into 1/2 inch (12 mm) strips	1	1
Yellow medium pepper, cut into 1/2 inch (12 mm) strips	1	1
Large onion, cut lengthwise into 8 wedges	1	1
Finely chopped pickled jalapeño peppers, drained	1 tbsp.	15 mL
Package of fajita seasoning mix	1 oz.	28 g
Water	1/4 cup	60 mL
Medium flour tortillas (8 inch, 20 cm, diameter)	10	10
Medium avocado, diced	1	1
Lemon juice	2 tsp.	10 mL
Light sour cream	2/3 cup	150 mL
Grated jalapeño Monterey Jack cheese	2/3 cup	150 mL
Medium tomato, seeded and diced	1	1
Shredded lettuce, lightly packed	1 cup	250 mL

Combine first 5 ingredients in 3 1/2 quart (3.5 L) slow cooker.

Combine seasoning mix and water in small dish. Add to slow cooker. Cover. Cook on Low for 5 to 6 hours or on High for 2 1/2 to 3 hours until beef is tender.

Strain beef and vegetables, reserving liquid for another purpose. Spoon about 1/2 cup (125 mL) beef mixture onto each tortilla.

Combine avocado and lemon juice in small bowl. Spoon avocado mixture over beef mixture on each tortilla.

Layer remaining 4 ingredients over avocado. Fold bottom edge up and over filling. Fold in sides, leaving top open. Secure with wooden pick if desired. Makes 10 fajitas.

1 fajita: 358 Calories; 16.5 g Total Fat (4.8 g Mono, 1.1 g Poly, 5.5 g Sat); 56 mg Cholesterol; 32 g Carbohydrate; 3 g Fibre; 22 g Protein; 698 mg Sodium

CHOICES: 1 1/2 Grains & Starches; 1/2 Vegetables; 2 Meat & Alternatives; 1 Fats

Pictured on page 72.

Squash and Lentil Soup

A delicious, thick and hearty soup with a velvety smooth texture.

Canola oil	2 tsp.	10 mL
Chopped onion	2 cups	500 mL
Garlic cloves, minced	2	2
(or 1/2 tsp., 2 mL, powder)		
Finely grated ginger root	1 tsp.	5 mL
(or 1/4 tsp., 1 mL, ground ginger)		
Curry powder	1 tbsp.	15 mL
Red lentils	1 1/2 cups	375 mL
Low-sodium prepared chicken broth	6 cups	1.5 L
Chopped butternut squash	5 cups	1.25 L
(about 1 1/2 lbs., 680 g)		
Salt	1/2 tsp.	2 mL
Low-fat plain yogurt	1/3 cup	75 mL

Heat canola oil in large frying pan on medium. Add next 3 ingredients. Cook for 5 to 10 minutes, stirring often, until onion is softened.

Add curry powder. Heat and stir for 1 to 2 minutes until fragrant. Transfer to 5 quart (5 L) slow cooker.

Add next 4 ingredients. Stir. Cover. Cook on Low for 6 to 8 hours or on High for 3 to 4 hours until lentils and squash are tender. Cool slightly. Process lentil mixture in blender or food processor until smooth (see Safety Tip). Return to slow cooker.

Add yogurt. Stir. Cover. Cook on High for about 15 minutes until heated through. Makes 9 1/2 cups (2.4 L). Serves 6.

1 serving: 325 Calories; 3.1 g Total Fat (1.0 g Mono, 0.6 g Poly, 0.3 g Sat); 5.8 mg Cholesterol; 60 g Carbohydrate; 12 g Fibre; 18 g Protein; 820 mg Sodium

CHOICES: 1 1/2 Grains & Starches; 5 Vegetables; 2 Meat & Alternatives

Safety Tip: Follow manufacturer's instructions for processing hot liquids.

Moroccan Chicken

Serve this spicy dish with couscous or Spinach Mushroom Rice, page 93. You'll enjoy the full-flavoured, well-seasoned sauce.

Canola oil	2 tsp.	10 mL
Thinly sliced onion	2 cups	500 mL
Garlic cloves, minced	2	2
(or 1/2 tsp., 2 mL, powder)		
Finely grated ginger root	1/2 tsp.	2 mL
Ground cumin	1/2 tsp.	2 mL
Ground coriander	1/2 tsp.	2 mL
Chili powder	1/2 tsp.	2 mL
Boneless, skinless chicken thighs, halved	1 lb.	454 g
Salt	1/4 tsp.	1 mL
Cinnamon stick (4 inch, 10 cm)	1	1
Cardamom, bruised (see Tip, page 27)	6	6
or 1/4 tsp. (1 mL), ground		
Dry (or alcohol-free) white wine	1/2 cup	125 mL
Liquid honey	2 tbsp.	30 mL
Orange juice	1/4 cup	60 mL
Cornstarch	2 tsp.	10 mL
Slivered almonds, toasted	3 tbsp.	50 mL
(see Tip, page 97)		

Heat canola oil in large frying pan on medium. Add next 3 ingredients. Cook for 5 to 10 minutes, stirring often, until onion is softened and starting to brown.

Add next 3 ingredients. Heat and stir for 1 to 2 minutes until fragrant. Transfer to 3 1/2 to 4 quart (3.5 to 4 L) slow cooker.

Add next 6 ingredients. Stir. Cover. Cook on Low for 7 to 8 hours or on High for 3 1/2 to 4 hours until chicken is no longer pink inside.

Stir orange juice into cornstarch in small bowl until smooth. Stir into chicken mixture. Cover. Cook on High for about 15 minutes until thickened. Remove and discard cinnamon stick and cardamom. Makes 3 cups (750 mL). Serves 4.

(continued on next page)

Orange Chicken

Tender chicken in an orange-flavoured sauce. Serve with rice and salad. This is a child-friendly entrée—no onions, no green bits and lots of those little orange pieces!

Hot water	1/4 cup	60 mL
Chicken bouillon powder	1 tsp.	5 mL
Can of unsweetened mandarin orange segments in juice	10 oz.	284 mL
Orange juice	1 cup	250 mL
Finely chopped fresh rosemary (or 1/2 tsp., 2 mL, dried, crushed)	2 tsp.	10 mL
Lemon pepper	1 tsp.	5 mL
Paprika	1/2 tsp.	2 mL
Bone-in chicken parts, skin removed	3 lbs.	1.4 kg
Water	2 tbsp.	30 mL
Cornstarch	2 tbsp.	30 mL

Stir hot water into bouillon powder in small bowl until dissolved.

Drain juice from oranges into same bowl. Set orange segments aside.

Add next 4 ingredients to juice mixture. Stir. Pour into 3 1/2 quart (3.5 L) slow cooker.

Add chicken, pressing down into juice mixture. Cover. Cook on Low for 7 to 8 hours or on High for 3 1/2 to 4 hours until chicken is no longer pink inside.

Stir water into cornstarch in small bowl until smooth. Add to slow cooker. Stir. Cover. Cook on High for about 15 minutes until sauce is thickened. Add orange segments. Stir. Serves 4.

Mustard Dill Halibut

A sweet, tangy sauce coats these moist, tender fish steaks. Serve with Crunchy Rice Salad, page 97, and Pea Medley, page 110.

Maple syrup	1/4 cup	60 mL
Dijon mustard (with whole seeds)	2 tbsp.	30 mL
Chopped fresh dill	2 tbsp.	30 mL
(or 1 1/2 tsp., 7 mL, dried)		
Lemon juice	2 tbsp.	30 mL
Garlic clove, minced	1	1
(or 1/4 tsp., 1 mL, powder)		
Salt	1/2 tsp.	2 mL
Small halibut steaks	4	4
(about 1 1/2 lbs., 680 g, total)		

Combine first 6 ingredients in small bowl.

Place halibut in shallow dish. Pour maple syrup mixture over fish. Turn until coated. Marinate in refrigerator for 3 to 5 hours, turning several times. Drain and discard marinade. Preheat greased two-sided grill for 5 minutes. Arrange fish on grill. Close lid. Cook for 5 to 8 minutes until fish flakes easily when tested with fork. Serves 4.

1 serving: 209 Calories; 4.1 g Total Fat (1.3 g Mono, 1.3 g Poly, 0.6 g Sat); 54 mg Cholesterol; 5 g Carbohydrate; trace Fibre; 36 g Protein; 203 mg Sodium

CHOICES: 5 Meat & Alternatives

Pictured on page 36.

MUSTARD DILL SALMON: Omit halibut. Use same amount of salmon fillet.

1 serving: 326 Calories; 18.0 g Total Fat (7.5 g Mono, 4.8 g Poly, 5.3 g Sat); 85 mg Cholesterol; 5 g Carbohydrate; trace Fibre; 34 g Protein; 192 mg Sodium

CHOICES: 5 Meat & Alternatives

Orange Teriyaki Fish

Basa is a tender, moist white fish that absorbs marinade flavours easily. Serve with Mashed Sweet Potatoes, page 103.

Soy sauce	2 tbsp.	30 mL
Frozen concentrated orange juice, thawed	2 tbsp.	30 mL
Corn syrup	1 tbsp.	15 mL
Finely grated ginger root	1 tsp.	5 mL
Lemon pepper	1/2 tsp.	2 mL
Basa fillets, any small bones removed (about 1 1/4 lbs., 560 g)	4	4

Combine first 5 ingredients in small cup.

Arrange fish, in single layer, in ungreased 9 x 13 inch (23 x 33 cm) pan. Spoon marinade over fish. Turn until coated. Cover. Marinate in refrigerator for 30 minutes. Preheat greased two-sided grill for 5 minutes. Place fish on grill. Close lid. Cook for about 4 minutes until fish flakes easily when tested with fork. Serves 4.

1 serving: 145 Calories; 5.7 g Total Fat (0 g Mono, 0 g Poly, 2.1 g Sat); 64 mg Cholesterol; 4 g Carbohydrate; 0 g Fibre; 19 g Protein; 472 mg Sodium

CHOICES: 2 1/2 Meat & Alternatives

Paré Pointer

Robots have good posture—they sit bolt upright

Pesto Chicken Wraps

These attractive grilled tortillas are fully stuffed with fresh asparagus, peppers and chicken. Use a store-bought roasted chicken for this recipe to make it quicker and easier. Serve with a tomato and basil salad or Oven-Fried Vegetables, page 111.

Fresh asparagus spears, trimmed of tough ends	6	6
Boiling water		
Sun-dried tomato pesto	1/3 cup	75 mL
Fat-free mayonnaise	2 tbsp.	30 mL
Flour tortillas (10 inch, 25 cm, diameter)	2	2
Chopped cooked chicken	2 cups	500 mL
Coarsely chopped roasted red peppers, blotted dry	1/2 cup	125 mL
Thinly sliced fresh white mushrooms	1/2 cup	125 mL

Cook asparagus in small amount of boiling water in frying pan on medium-high for about 2 minutes until tender-crisp. Remove to paper towel to drain well.

Combine pesto and mayonnaise in small bowl. Spread over tortillas.

Layer chicken, red pepper, asparagus and mushrooms along centre of each tortilla. Fold sides of tortilla over filling. Roll up from bottom to enclose filling. Preheat greased two-sided grill for 5 minutes. Place wraps on grill. Close lid. Cook for about 5 minutes until crisp and browned. To serve, cut each wrap in half diagonally. Serves 4.

1 serving: 378 Calories; 14.3 g Total Fat (5.5 g Mono, 3.2 g Poly, 3.8 g Sat); 77 mg Cholesterol; 29 g Carbohydrate; 2 g Fibre; 29 g Protein; 869 mg Sodium

CHOICES: 1 Grains & Starches; 1 Vegetables; 3 Meat & Alternatives

Grilled Pork Mushrooms

Excellent served with Maple Butternut Squash, page 104, and a drizzle of
Spicy Roasted Pepper Sauce, page 113.

Lean ground pork	8 oz.	225 g
Garlic clove, minced (or 1/4 – 1/2 tsp., 1 – 2 mL, powder)	1 – 2	1 – 2
Green onions, thinly sliced	2	2
Low-sodium soy sauce	1 tbsp.	15 mL
Finely chopped fresh parsley (or 3/4 tsp., 4 mL, flakes)	1 tbsp.	15 mL
Dry sherry	2 tsp.	10 mL
Egg white (large)	1	1
Dried crushed chilies	1/4 tsp.	1 mL
Pepper	1/4 tsp.	1 mL
Portobello mushrooms (5 inch, 12.5 cm, diameter), stems removed	4	4
Sesame seeds	1 tsp.	5 mL
Paprika	1/4 tsp.	1 mL

Combine first 9 ingredients in medium bowl.

Scrape black "gills" from underside of mushrooms with spoon and discard. Spoon pork mixture into mushroom cavities. Spread evenly.

Sprinkle with sesame seeds and paprika. Preheat greased two-sided grill for 5 minutes. Arrange mushrooms, stuffed-side up, on grill. Close lid. Cook for about 5 minutes until pork is no longer pink. Makes 4 stuffed mushrooms. Serves 2.

1 serving: 385 Calories; 25.1 g Total Fat (10.7 g Mono, 2.2 g Poly, 8.9 g Sat); 82 mg Cholesterol; 12 g Carbohydrate; 3 g Fibre; 26 g Protein; 376 mg Sodium

CHOICES: 1 Vegetables; 3 Meat & Alternatives

Apricot-Glazed Chicken

Moist chicken with a tangy glaze. Serve with Fluffy Garlic Potatoes, page 88, and Asparagus and Mushrooms, page 109.

Can of apricots in light syrup, drained	14 oz.	398 mL
Brown sugar, packed	1 tbsp.	15 mL
Lemon juice	2 tsp.	10 mL
Garlic chili sauce	1 tsp.	5 mL
Boneless, skinless chicken thighs	1 lb.	454 g

Process first 4 ingredients in blender or food processor until smooth. Pour into large resealable freezer bag.

Add chicken. Seal bag. Turn until coated. Marinate in refrigerator for at least 24 hours, turning several times. Remove chicken from bag. Transfer remaining apricot mixture to small saucepan. Bring to a boil. Boil for about 5 minutes, stirring often, until reduced and slightly thickened. Preheat greased two-sided grill for 5 minutes. Arrange chicken on grill. Close lid. Cook for 5 to 7 minutes until browned and no longer pink inside. Remove to serving plate. Drizzle apricot mixture over chicken. Serves 4.

1 serving: 261 Calories; 8.6 g Total Fat (3.3 g Mono, 2.0 g Poly, 2.4 g Sat); 74 mg Cholesterol; 25 g Carbohydrate; 3 g Fibre; 21 g Protein; 114 mg Sodium

CHOICES: 1 1/2 Fruits; 3 Meat & Alternatives

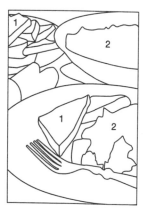

1. Mushroom Polenta, page 99
2. Chicken Cacciatore, page 48

Props courtesy of: Danesco Inc.

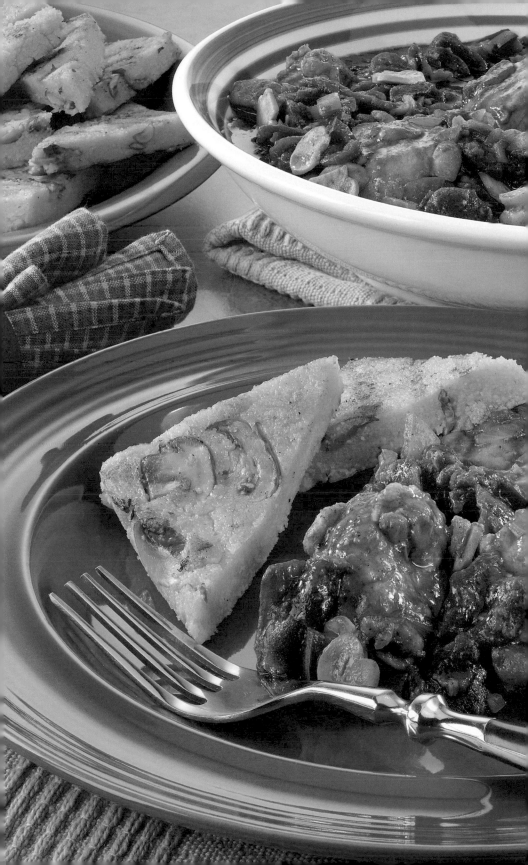

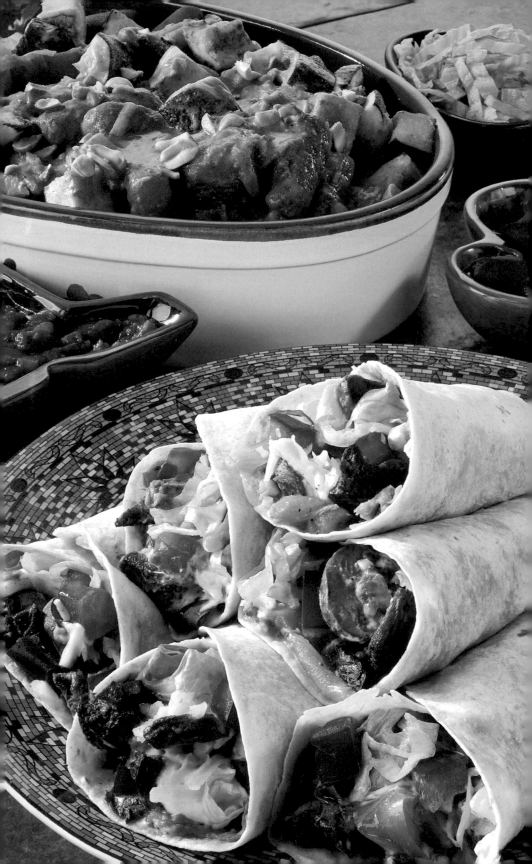

Peppered Lamb

Tender lamb chops with a hint of garlic and mint flavour in the coating. These are so easy and flavourful that they will become a favourite. Serve with Creamed Veggie Spaghetti, page 94, and Zucchini Pepper Combo, page 105.

Finely chopped fresh mint	2 tbsp.	30 mL
(or 1 1/2 tsp., 7 mL, dried)		
Olive (or canola) oil	1 tbsp.	15 mL
Garlic cloves, minced	2	2
(or 1/2 tsp., 2 mL, powder)		
Pepper	1/2 tsp.	2 mL
Lean lamb loin chops (about 1 1/4 – 1 1/2 lbs., 560 – 680 g, total), about 1 1/4 inches (3 cm), thick	8	8

Combine first 4 ingredients in small dish.

Spread mint mixture over both sides of each lamb chop. Let stand on plate at room temperature for 15 minutes. Preheat greased two-sided grill for 5 minutes. Arrange chops on grill. Close lid. Cook for 8 to 10 minutes until desired doneness. Remove to plate. Tent with foil. Let stand for 10 minutes before serving. Makes 8 lamb chops. Serves 4.

1 serving: 292 Calories; 22.4 g Total Fat (10.4 g Mono, 1.9 g Poly, 8.6 g Sat); 82 mg Cholesterol; 1 g Carbohydrate; trace Fibre; 21 g Protein; 64 mg Sodium

CHOICES: 3 Meat & Alternatives; 1/2 Fats

Pictured on page 36.

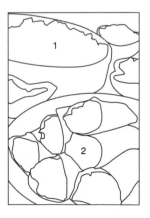

1. Peanut Butter Chicken, page 60
2. Slow Cooker Fajitas, page 62

Props courtesy of: Sears Canada

Grilled Chicken and Salsa

Lightly spiced chicken and bright, colourful salsa are a perfect match. Reserve some salsa for Beef and Rice Lettuce Wraps, page 76.

Lime juice	2 tbsp.	30 mL
Dried crushed chilies	1 tsp.	5 mL
Granulated sugar	1 tsp.	5 mL
Ground cinnamon	3/4 tsp.	4 mL
Ground cumin	1/2 tsp.	2 mL
Ground coriander	1/2 tsp.	2 mL
Garlic cloves, minced	2	2
(or 1/2 tsp., 2 mL, powder)		
Boneless, skinless chicken breast halves, flattened evenly (see Note)	1 lb.	454 g
FRESH CORN SALSA		
Medium corncobs	2	2
Medium tomatoes, seeds removed, chopped	3	3
Can of black beans, rinsed and drained	19 oz.	540 mL
Finely chopped celery	1/2 cup	125 mL
Thinly sliced green onion	1/2 cup	125 mL
Lime juice	1/3 cup	75 mL
Chopped fresh parsley	3 tbsp.	50 mL
Olive oil	2 tsp.	10 mL
Ground cumin	1/4 tsp.	1 mL
Hot pepper sauce	1/4 tsp.	1 mL
Garlic clove, minced	1	1
(or 1/4 tsp., 1 mL, powder)		

Combine first 7 ingredients in large shallow dish.

Add chicken. Turn until coated. Cover. Marinate in refrigerator for at least 8 hours or overnight, turning several times.

(continued on next page)

Fresh Corn Salsa: Preheat electric grill for 5 minutes or gas barbecue to high. Cook corncobs on greased grill for about 15 minutes, turning often, until corn is tender and browned. Let stand until cool enough to handle. Place cob, 1 end down, on cutting board. Run knife down length of cob, cutting off kernels. Put kernels into medium bowl. Discard cob. Repeat with second cob. Add next 4 ingredients to corn. Stir.

Combine next 6 ingredients in jar with tight-fitting lid. Shake well. Drizzle over corn mixture. Toss well. Makes 5 1/2 cups (1.4 L) salsa. Reserve 3 1/2 cups (875 mL) salsa in airtight container in refrigerator to use for Beef and Rice Lettuce Wraps, page 76. Remove chicken. Discard any remaining marinade from dish. Preheat electric grill for 5 minutes or gas barbecue to medium. Cook chicken on greased grill for about 5 minutes per side until no longer pink inside. Cut diagonally into 1/4 inch (6 mm) slices. Serve remaining salsa with grilled chicken. Serves 4.

1 serving: 202 Calories; 3.2 g Total Fat (0.9 g Mono, 0.8 g Poly, 0.5 g Sat); 66 mg Cholesterol; 12 g Carbohydrate; 3 g Fibre; 30 g Protein; 221 mg Sodium

CHOICES: 1/2 Grains & Starches; 4 Meat & Alternatives

Note: Gently pound thicker parts of chicken pieces with a meat mallet or rolling pin just until uniform thickness.

To Make Ahead: Marinate chicken and make salsa, omitting corn, the night before. Grill chicken and corn on electric grill or gas barbecue the next day. Add corn to salsa.

Kid-Friendly Idea: Omit dried crushed chilies and reduce strong spices by half.

Paré Pointer

Cross a pony with a 25-cent piece and you'll have a quarter horse.

Beef and Rice Lettuce Wraps

Moist beef, beans and rice fill large, fresh lettuce leaves. Fun to eat and mild-flavoured for kids.

Olive oil	1 tsp.	5 mL
Extra-lean ground beef	1/2 lb.	225 g
Chopped onion	1/2 cup	125 mL
Reserved Fresh Corn Salsa (from Grilled Chicken and Salsa, page 74), plus accumulated juice	3 1/2 cups	875 mL
Vegetable cocktail juice	1 cup	250 mL
Long grain white rice	2/3 cup	150 mL
Large lettuce leaves (butter, green leaf, red leaf or iceberg varieties), see Note	16 – 20	16 – 20

Heat olive oil in large saucepan on medium. Add beef and onion. Scramble-fry for about 5 minutes until beef is no longer pink and onion is softened.

Add salsa and cocktail juice. Bring to a boil. Add rice. Stir. Reduce heat to medium-low. Cover. Simmer for 15 to 20 minutes until rice is tender and liquid is absorbed. Remove from heat. Spoon into 4 serving bowls.

To serve, spoon 3 to 4 tbsp. (50 to 60 mL) rice mixture into centre of each lettuce leaf. Fold sides in and bottom up to enclose. Serves 4.

1 serving: 333 Calories; 6.5 g Total Fat (2.8 g Mono, 1.3 g Poly, 1.1 g Sat); 30 mg Cholesterol; 49 g Carbohydrate; 7 g Fibre; 20 g Protein; 451 mg Sodium

CHOICES: 2 Grains & Starches; 2 Meat & Alternatives; 1/2 Fats

Note: Soft lettuce varieties like butter and leaf are much easier to fold around filling. Iceberg lettuce, however, gives a cool, crisp crunch in contrast to the warm, soft filling. All of these lettuce varieties are nutritionally similar, so you can substitute whichever you desire without affecting carbs or Choices values.

Roasted Garlic Pork Supper

Pork is infused with a delicious roasted garlic flavour. Serve with unsweetened applesauce in place of traditional gravy. Reserve half of roast for Quick Pork With Noodles, page 78.

Pork loin roast	2 1/4 lbs.	1 kg
Garlic cloves, halved lengthwise	6	6
Liquid honey	1 tbsp.	15 mL
Paprika	1 tsp.	5 mL
Dry mustard	1 tsp.	5 mL
Pepper	1 tsp.	5 mL
Whole baby carrots	2 cups	500 mL
Small onions (root ends left intact), quartered lengthwise	3	3
Red baby potatoes, halved	1 lb.	454 g
Pepper	1/4 tsp.	1 mL
Chopped fresh parsley	1 tbsp.	15 mL

Cut 12 small Xs in top of roast. Insert half garlic clove into each X.

Combine next 4 ingredients in small dish. Spread over roast. Place in greased medium roasting pan.

Arrange next 3 ingredients around roast. Sprinkle with second amount of pepper. Cover. Cook in 325°F (160°C) oven for 1 1/2 to 2 hours until carrots are tender and meat thermometer inserted into thickest part of roast reads 155°F (68°C) for medium or until desired doneness. Cover with foil. Let stand for 10 minutes. Internal temperature should rise to at least 160°F (70°C). Slice half of roast, reserving remaining roast for Quick Pork With Noodles, page 78. Arrange pork slices and vegetables on platter.

Sprinkle with parsley. Serves 4.

1 serving: 354 Calories; 7.8 g Total Fat (3.4 g Mono, 0.7 g Poly, 2.6 g Sat); 81 mg Cholesterol; 38 g Carbohydrate; 4 g Fibre; 32 g Protein; 89 mg Sodium

CHOICES: 1 Grains & Starches; 2 Vegetables; 4 Meat & Alternatives

Kid-Friendly Idea: Omit garlic and reduce mustard.

Quick Pork With Noodles

A colourful medley of pasta and pork strips.

Hard margarine (or butter), softened	2 tsp.	10 mL
Finely chopped onion	1/2 cup	125 mL
Sliced fresh white mushrooms	1 1/2 cups	375 mL
Pepper	1/4 tsp.	1 mL
Green onions, thinly sliced	2	2
Finely chopped red pepper	1/4 cup	60 mL
Can of skim evaporated milk	13 1/2 oz.	385 mL
All-purpose flour	2 tbsp.	30 mL
Reserved pork (from Roasted Garlic Pork Supper, page 77), cut into thin strips	2 cups	500 mL
Light herb cream cheese	3 tbsp.	50 mL
Chopped fresh parsley (or 1 1/2 tsp., 7 mL, flakes)	2 tbsp.	30 mL
Balsamic vinegar	1 tsp.	5 mL
Boiling water	12 cups	3 L
Salt	1 tbsp.	15 mL
Package of large yolk-free broad noodles	12 oz.	340 g
Finely chopped fresh parsley	1 tbsp.	15 mL

Melt margarine in large non-stick frying pan on medium. Add next 3 ingredients. Cook for about 10 minutes, stirring often, until onion is softened and liquid is evaporated.

Add green onion and red pepper. Stir.

Stir evaporated milk into flour in small bowl until smooth. Add to onion mixture. Stir. Heat and stir on medium until boiling and slightly thickened.

Add next 4 ingredients. Heat and stir until cheese is melted and pork is heated through. Keep warm.

(continued on next page)

Combine boiling water and salt in large pot or Dutch oven. Add noodles. Cook, uncovered, for about 10 minutes, stirring occasionally, until tender but firm. Drain. Return to pot. Add pork mixture. Toss until coated. Transfer to serving bowl. Makes 9 1/2 cups (2.4 L).

Garnish with parsley. Serves 6.

1 serving: 468 Calories; 9.2 g Total Fat (3.4 g Mono, 0.8 g Poly, 3.1 g Sat); 71 mg Cholesterol; 57 g Carbohydrate; 4 g Fibre; 36 g Protein; 179 mg Sodium

CHOICES: 2 1/2 Grains & Starches; 1/2 Milk & Alternatives; 2 Meat & Alternatives

---

Paré Pointer

The teacher asked for "denial" in a sentence. The student wrote about a river in Egypt.

Basic Beef Stew

Tender beef with honey and mint flavours, and a warm, pleasant spiciness. Serve with cooling plain yogurt and Easy Coucous, page 92. Reserve half of stew for Spicy Beef Pie, page 81.

Stewing beef, trimmed of fat	2 lbs.	900 g
All-purpose flour	1/4 cup	60 mL
Canola oil	2 tsp.	10 mL
Canola oil	2 tsp.	10 mL
Chopped onion	2 cups	500 mL
Garlic cloves, minced	2	2
(or 1/2 tsp., 2 mL, powder)		
Ground cumin	1 tsp.	5 mL
Ground coriander	1 tsp.	5 mL
Ground ginger	1 tsp.	5 mL
Dried crushed chilies	1 tsp.	5 mL
Low-sodium prepared beef broth	1 1/2 cups	375 mL
Medium carrots, chopped	2	2
Chopped celery	3/4 cup	175 mL
Liquid honey	1 tbsp.	15 mL
Chopped fresh mint	2 tbsp.	30 mL

Combine beef and flour in plastic bag. Toss until coated. Shake excess flour from beef. Transfer beef to plate. Discard any remaining flour. Heat first amount of canola oil in large non-stick frying pan on medium. Cook beef, in 2 batches, until browned. Transfer to large pot or Dutch oven. Cover to keep warm.

Heat second amount of canola oil in same pan on medium. Add onion and garlic. Cook for 5 to 10 minutes, stirring often, scraping any browned bits from pan, until onion is softened.

Add next 4 ingredients. Heat and stir for 1 to 2 minutes until fragrant.

Add 1/2 cup (125 mL) broth to onion mixture. Stir. Add to beef. Add remaining broth, carrot and celery. Bring to a boil on medium-high. Reduce heat to medium-low. Cover. Cook for about 1 1/2 hours until beef is tender. Simmer, uncovered, for 15 to 20 minutes until sauce is slightly thickened. Makes about 5 cups (1.25 L) stew. Reserve half of stew and store in airtight container in refrigerator to use for Spicy Beef Pie, page 81.

(continued on next page)

Add honey and mint to remaining stew. Heat and stir on medium until heated through. Makes 2 1/2 cups (625 mL). Serves 4.

1 serving: 305 Calories; 17.2 g Total Fat (7.7 g Mono, 1.3 g Poly, 5.9 g Sat); 70 mg Cholesterol; 15 g Carbohydrate; 2 g Fibre; 22 g Protein; 84 mg Sodium

CHOICES: 1 Vegetables; 3 Meat & Alternatives; 1/2 Fats

Pictured on page 90.

Kid-Friendly Idea: Reduce spices by half and omit crushed chilies.

Spicy Beef Pie

Satisfying and crispy pastry "puffs" cover richly flavoured and tender beef stew. So easy to make this completely unique presentation.

Reserved stew (from Basic Beef Stew, page 80)	2 1/2 cups	625 mL
Phyllo pastry sheets, thawed according to package directions	8	8
Sesame seeds	2 tsp.	10 mL

Spread stew evenly in lightly greased 9 inch (23 cm) deep dish pie plate.

Spray 1 phyllo sheet with cooking spray. Bunch up loosely. Place on top of stew. Repeat with remaining phyllo sheets.

Lightly spray top of pie with cooking spray. Sprinkle with sesame seeds. Bake in 375°F (175°C) oven for 20 to 25 minutes until beef mixture is hot and pastry is lightly browned. Serves 4.

1 serving: 333 Calories; 15.6 g Total Fat (6.8 g Mono, 1.3 g Poly, 4.9 g Sat); 51 mg Cholesterol; 28 g Carbohydrate; 2 g Fibre; 19 g Protein; 247 mg Sodium

CHOICES: 1 1/2 Grains & Starches; 1 1/2 Meat & Alternatives; 1 Fats

Pictured on page 90.

Creamy Chicken Spaghetti

A perfectly coated creamy pasta. Reserve half of sauce for Garden Chicken Stew, page 83.

CHICKEN SAUCE

Canola oil	2 tsp.	10 mL
Boneless, skinless chicken thighs, quartered	2 lbs.	900 g
Canola oil	2 tsp.	10 mL
Leeks (white and tender green parts only), thinly sliced	2	2
Garlic cloves, minced (or 1 tsp., 5 mL, powder)	4	4
Sliced fresh white mushrooms	4 cups	1 L
All-purpose flour	1/4 cup	60 mL
Low-sodium prepared chicken broth	3 cups	750 mL
Dijon mustard (with whole seeds)	2 tbsp.	30 mL
Boiling water	12 cups	3 L
Salt	1 tsp.	5 mL
Spaghetti	12 oz.	340 g
Light sour cream	1/4 cup	60 mL
Chopped fresh basil (or 2 1/4 tsp., 11 mL, dried)	3 tbsp.	50 mL
Salt	1/4 tsp.	1 mL
Pepper	1/4 tsp.	1 mL

Chicken Sauce: Heat first amount of canola oil in large saucepan on medium-high. Cook chicken, in 2 to 3 batches, for about 3 minutes per side, stirring often, until lightly browned. Remove from saucepan. Cover to keep warm.

Heat second amount of canola oil in same saucepan on medium. Add next 3 ingredients. Cook for 5 to 10 minutes, stirring often, until leek is softened and mushrooms are browned.

Add flour. Heat and stir for 1 minute. Gradually stir in broth. Heat and stir on medium until boiling and thickened. Add mustard. Stir. Add chicken. Cook for about 15 minutes, stirring often, until chicken is tender. Makes 6 1/2 cups (1.6 L) sauce. Reserve half of sauce in airtight container in refrigerator to use for Garden Chicken Stew, page 83.

(continued on next page)

Combine boiling water and salt in large pot or Dutch oven. Add spaghetti. Cook, uncovered, for 10 to 12 minutes, stirring occasionally, until tender but firm. Drain. Return to same pot.

Add remaining 4 ingredients to remaining chicken mixture. Heat and stir on medium until heated through. Add to spaghetti. Toss until coated. Makes 7 cups (1.75 L). Serves 6.

1 serving: 375 Calories; 9.3 g Total Fat (3.0 g Mono, 1.8 g Poly, 2.2 g Sat); 54 mg Cholesterol; 48 g Carbohydrate; 2 g Fibre; 23 g Protein; 367 mg Sodium

CHOICES: 3 Grains & Starches; 2 Meat & Alternatives

Garden Chicken Stew

A hearty stew with a hint of lemon.

Reserved Chicken Sauce (from Creamy Chicken Spaghetti, page 82)	3 1/4 cups	800 mL
Medium peeled potatoes, chopped	2	2
Medium carrots, chopped	2	2
Low-sodium prepared chicken broth	1/2 cup	125 mL
Garlic clove, minced (or 1/4 tsp., 1 mL, powder)	1	1
Frozen peas	2/3 cup	150 mL
Chopped fresh parsley	3 tbsp.	50 mL
Finely grated lemon zest	1 tsp.	5 mL

Combine first 5 ingredients in large pot or Dutch oven. Bring to a boil on medium-high. Reduce heat to medium-low. Cover. Cook for about 20 minutes, stirring occasionally, until vegetables are tender.

Add peas. Heat and stir for about 5 minutes until heated through. Remove from heat.

Sprinkle parsley and lemon zest over top. Stir. Makes 5 1/2 cups (1.4 L). Serves 4.

1 serving: 276 Calories; 9.6 g Total Fat (3.9 g Mono, 2.2 g Poly, 2.2 g Sat); 65 mg Cholesterol; 26 g Carbohydrate; 4 g Fibre; 23 g Protein; 451 mg Sodium

CHOICES: 1 Vegetables; 2 Meat & Alternatives

Kid-Friendly Idea: Omit garlic, parsley and lemon zest.

Penne and Meat Sauce

A thick, hearty, full-bodied meat sauce. The oregano, garlic and wine flavours are distinct and blend nicely. Reserve half of sauce for Potato Beef Pie, page 85.

GROUND BEEF SAUCE

Canola oil	2 tsp.	10 mL
Chopped onion	2 cups	500 mL
Garlic cloves, minced	2	2
(or 1/2 tsp., 2 mL, powder)		
Extra-lean ground beef	2 lbs.	900 g
Can of diced tomatoes (with juice)	28 oz.	796 mL
Red (or alcohol-free) wine	1 cup	250 mL
Can of tomato paste	5 1/2 oz.	156 mL
Chopped fresh oregano	2 tbsp.	30 mL
(or 1 1/2 tsp., 7 mL, dried)		
Granulated sugar	1 tsp.	5 mL
Bay leaf	1	1
Salt, sprinkle		
Pepper	1/4 tsp.	1 mL
Boiling water	12 cups	3 L
Salt	1 tsp.	5 mL
Penne pasta	3 cups	750 mL

Ground Beef Sauce: Heat canola oil in large pot or Dutch oven on medium. Add onion and garlic. Cook for 5 to 10 minutes, stirring often, until onion is softened.

Add ground beef. Scramble-fry on medium-high for about 15 minutes until no pink remains.

Add next 8 ingredients. Stir. Bring to a boil. Reduce heat to medium-low. Cook, uncovered, for about 20 minutes, stirring occasionally, until sauce is thickened. Makes 7 cups (1.75 L) sauce. Reserve half of sauce in airtight container in refrigerator to use for Potato Beef Pie, page 85.

Combine boiling water and salt in large pot or Dutch oven. Add pasta. Cook, uncovered, for 10 to 12 minutes, stirring occasionally, until tender but firm. Drain. Transfer pasta to large serving bowl or individual bowls. Spoon remaining sauce over top. Serves 4.

1 serving: 541 Calories; 7.2 g Total Fat (2.7 g Mono, 0.9 g Poly, 1.6 g Sat); 60 mg Cholesterol; 78 g Carbohydrate; 5 g Fibre; 35 g Protein; 353 mg Sodium

CHOICES: 4 Grains & Starches; 2 Vegetables; 3 Meat & Alternatives

Potato Beef Pie

This Italian version of shepherd's pie is a great meal for everyone—warm and inviting.

MASHED POTATO TOPPING

Boiling water		
Salt	1/2 tsp.	2 mL
Peeled potatoes, chopped	2 lbs.	900 g
Milk	1 – 2 tbsp.	15 – 30 mL
Pepper	1/8 tsp.	0.5 mL

BEEF FILLING

Reserved Ground Beef Sauce (from Penne and Meat Sauce, page 84)	3 1/2 cups	875 mL
Frozen mixed vegetables, thawed	1 1/2 cups	375 mL
Ketchup	3 tbsp.	50 mL
Worcestershire sauce	2 tsp.	10 mL
Finely grated fresh Parmesan cheese	1/4 cup	60 mL
Chopped fresh parsley	1 tbsp.	15 mL

Mashed Potato Topping: Combine boiling water and salt in medium saucepan. Add potato. Cook on medium for about 15 minutes until tender. Drain. Mash potato until no lumps remain.

Add milk and pepper. Mix well.

Beef Filling: Combine first 4 ingredients in medium bowl. Transfer to greased 2 quart (2 L) casserole. Smooth top. Spread potato topping evenly over top.

Sprinkle with Parmesan cheese. Bake in 400°F (205°C) oven for about 30 minutes until heated through.

Sprinkle with parsley. Let stand for 10 minutes before serving. Serves 4.

1 serving: 378 Calories; 7.6 g Total Fat (1.8 g Mono, 0.6 g Poly, 3.2 g Sat); 49 mg Cholesterol; 59 g Carbohydrate; 6 g Fibre; 25 g Protein; 600 mg Sodium

CHOICES: 2 1/2 Grains & Starches; 1 Vegetables; 2 1/2 Meats & Alternatives

Grilled Pork Sandwiches

A tasty pork sandwich that will become a favourite. Reserve half of marinade and two cutlets for Spinach and Pork Salad, page 87.

ZESTY MARINADE

Lemon juice	1/2 cup	125 mL
Chopped fresh parsley	1/3 cup	75 mL
(or 3 1/2 tsp., 17 mL, flakes)		
Olive oil	2 tbsp.	30 mL
Liquid honey	1 tbsp.	15 mL
Finely grated lemon zest	2 tsp.	10 mL
Chili paste (sambal oelek)	2 tsp.	10 mL
Garlic cloves, minced	2	2
(or 1/2 tsp., 2 mL, powder)		
Pepper	1/2 tsp.	2 mL
Lean pork cutlets	4	4
Sun-dried tomatoes in oil, drained and finely chopped	2 tbsp.	30 mL
Low-fat mayonnaise	2 tbsp.	30 mL
Crusty bread loaf (such as ciabatta), split	1	1
Fresh spinach leaves, lightly packed, torn	1/2 cup	125 mL
Sliced fresh white mushrooms	1/2 cup	125 mL

Zesty Marinade: Combine first 8 ingredients in large bowl.

Add pork cutlets. Turn until coated. Cover. Marinate in refrigerator for at least 15 minutes. Preheat electric grill for 5 minutes or gas barbecue to medium. Cook 2 cutlets on greased grill for 3 to 4 minutes per side until tender. Reserve remaining 2 cutlets in marinade in refrigerator to use for Spinach and Pork Salad, page 87.

Combine sun-dried tomatoes and mayonnaise in small bowl.

Broil bread loaf, cut sides up, until lightly toasted. Spread mayonnaise mixture onto bottom half of bread loaf.

Layer cutlets, spinach and mushrooms over mayonnaise. Cover with top of bread loaf. Cut crosswise into 4 sandwiches.

1 sandwich: 416 Calories; 16.2 g Total Fat (7.0 g Mono, 1.4 g Poly, 5.3 g Sat); 64 mg Cholesterol; 40 g Carbohydrate; 2 g Fibre; 26 g Protein; 632 mg Sodium

CHOICES: 2 Grains & Starches; 3 Meat & Alternatives; 1 Fats

Pictured on page 107 and on back cover.

Spinach and Pork Salad

A large meal salad with a tart lemon flavour and a lingering chili heat.

Reserved pork cutlets in Zesty Marinade (from Grilled Pork Sandwiches, page 86)	2	2
Fresh spinach leaves, lightly packed	4 cups	1 L
Can of chickpeas, rinsed and drained	19 oz.	540 mL
Blanched fresh (or frozen) whole green beans, trimmed (see Note)	1 1/2 cups	375 mL
Roma (plum) tomatoes, quartered lengthwise	4	4
Thinly sliced red onion	1/2 cup	125 mL
LEMON CHILI DRESSING		
Lemon juice	1/4 cup	60 mL
Chopped fresh parsley (or 1 1/2 tsp., 7 mL, dried)	2 tbsp.	30 mL
Olive oil	1 tbsp.	15 mL
Chili paste (sambal oelek)	1 tsp.	5 mL
Salt	1/4 tsp.	1 mL

Preheat electric grill for 5 minutes or gas barbecue to medium. Remove cutlets from marinade. Discard any remaining marinade. Cook cutlets on greased grill for 3 to 4 minutes per side until tender. Cut crosswise into thin strips.

Combine next 5 ingredients in large bowl. Add pork. Toss.

Lemon Chili Dressing: Process all 5 ingredients in blender or food processor until smooth. Makes about 1/3 cup (75 mL) dressing. Drizzle over salad. Toss. Makes 12 cups (3 L) salad. Serves 4 to 6.

1 serving: 772 Calories; 24.9 g Total Fat (11.1 g Mono, 5.6 g Poly, 5.3 g Sat); 63 mg Cholesterol; 94 g Carbohydrate; 26 g Fibre; 47 g Protein; 345 mg Sodium

CHOICES: 4 Grains & Starches; 1 Vegetables; 7 Meat & Alternatives; 1 Fats

Pictured on page 107 and on back cover.

Note: To blanch beans, add to boiling water in large saucepan. Cook for 3 minutes. Drain. Immediately plunge into ice water for about 10 minutes until cold. Drain well.

Kid-Friendly Idea: Substitute same amount of iceberg lettuce for the spinach. Reduce or omit chili paste.

Fluffy Garlic Potatoes

Fluffy mashed potatoes with lots of fresh parsley flecks and a tangy garlic flavour. A wonderful addition to any grilled or roasted entrée.

Water		
Salt	1/4 tsp.	1 mL
Peeled medium baking potatoes, quartered	4	4
Low-fat plain yogurt	3 tbsp.	50 mL
Chopped fresh parsley	2 tbsp.	30 mL
(or 1 1/2 tsp., 7 mL, flakes)		
Garlic clove, minced	1	1
(or 1/4 tsp., 1 mL, powder)		
Pepper	1/4 tsp.	1 mL

Combine water and salt in medium saucepan on medium-high. Add potato. Cook for about 20 minutes until tender. Drain. Mash well.

Add remaining 4 ingredients. Stir with fork until fluffy and no lumps remain. Makes 2 1/2 cups (625 mL).

1/2 cup (125 mL): 87 Calories; 0.1 g Total Fat (0 g Mono, 0 g Poly, 0.1 g Sat); 0.6 mg Cholesterol; 22 g Carbohydrate; 2.5 g Fibre; 3.7 g Protein; 65 mg Sodium

CHOICES: 1 Grains & Starches

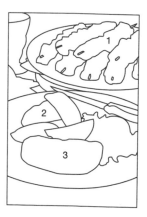

1. Pepper Pork Skewers, page 38
2. Crispy Spiced Potatoes, page 100
3. Lemon Garlic Steaks, page 16

Props courtesy of: Pier 1 Imports
Wiltshire®

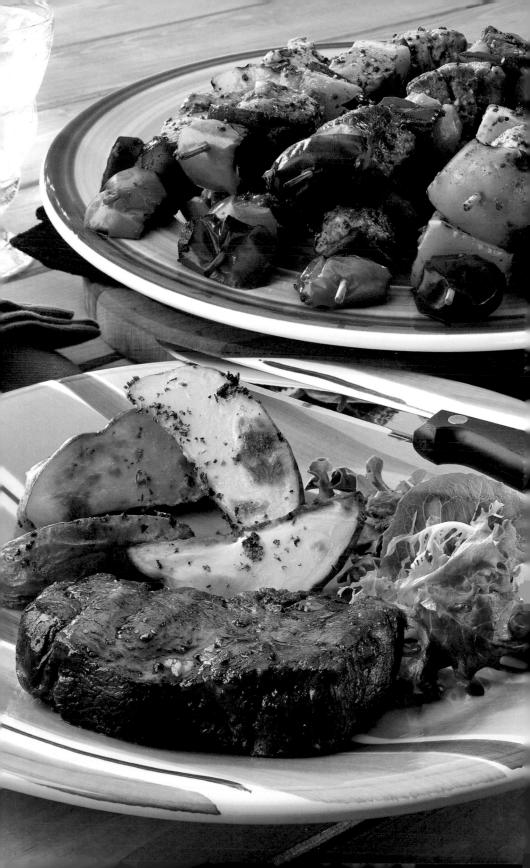

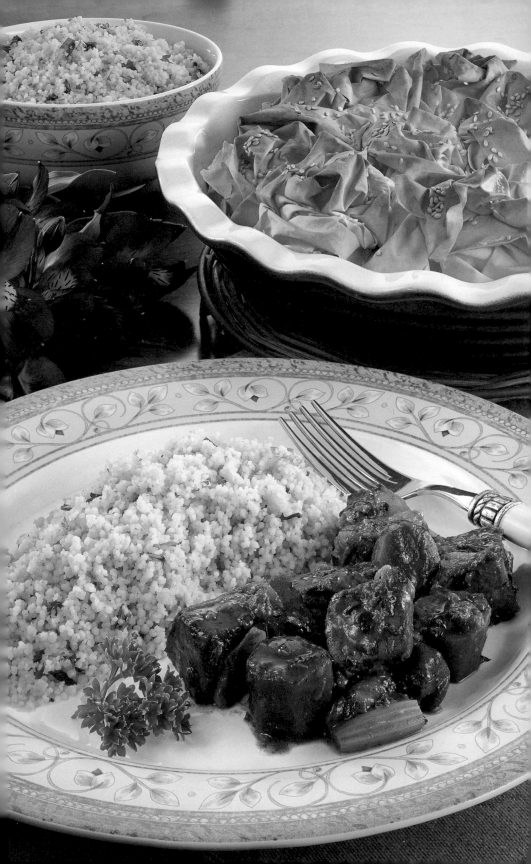

Pasta Salad

A great balance of flavours that taste like summer.

LEMON DRESSING		
Low-fat mayonnaise	1/3 cup	75 mL
Chopped fresh parsley	3 tbsp.	50 mL
(or 2 1/4 tsp., 11 mL, flakes)		
Lemon juice	1 – 2 tbsp.	15 – 30 mL
Liquid honey	1 tbsp.	15 mL
Garlic clove, minced	1	1
Pepper	1/4 tsp.	1 mL
Cooked penne pasta	2 cups	500 mL
Medium tomatoes, seeds removed, chopped	2	2
Chopped green onion	1/2 cup	125 mL
Can of artichoke hearts, drained and chopped	14 oz.	398 mL

Lemon Dressing: Combine first 6 ingredients in large bowl. Makes 1/2 cup (125 mL) dressing.

Add remaining 4 ingredients. Toss until coated. Makes 6 cups (1.5 L).

1/2 cup (125 mL): 108 Calories; 1.3 g Total Fat (0 g Mono, 0 g Poly, 0.2 g Sat); 0 mg Cholesterol; 20 g Carbohydrate; 1 g Fibre; 3 g Protein; 142 mg Sodium

CHOICES: 1 Grains & Starches

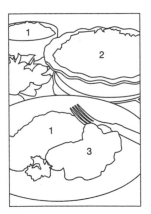

1. Easy Couscous, page 92
2. Spicy Beef Pie, page 81
3. Basic Beef Stew, page 80

Props courtesy of: Pfaltzgraff Canada
Casa Bugatti
Canhome Global

Easy Couscous

Fluffy, golden couscous speckled with green onion and fresh parsley. Subtle cumin and ginger spices add an exotic flavour. Makes a delicious side dish for Blackened Snapper, page 23, or Marinated Halibut Skewers, page 29.

Olive oil	1 tsp.	5 mL
Chopped green onion	1 cup	250 mL
Ground cumin	1/2 tsp.	2 mL
Ground ginger	1/2 tsp.	2 mL
Garlic clove, minced (or 1/4 tsp., 1 mL, powder)	1	1
Liquid honey	1 tbsp.	15 mL
Low-sodium prepared chicken broth	2 cups	500 mL
Whole-wheat couscous	2 cups	500 mL
Olive oil	2 tsp.	10 mL
Chopped fresh parsley (or 2 1/4 tsp., 11 mL, flakes)	3 tbsp.	50 mL
Pepper	1/4 tsp.	1 mL

Heat first amount of olive oil in medium saucepan on medium. Add next 4 ingredients. Cook and stir for about 3 minutes until green onion is softened.

Add honey. Heat and stir for about 30 seconds until green onion is coated.

Add broth. Bring to a boil. Add couscous and second amount of olive oil. Stir. Cover. Remove from heat. Let stand for 5 minutes without lifting lid. Fluff with fork.

Stir in parsley and pepper. Makes 5 1/2 cups (1.4 L).

1/2 cup (125 mL): 99 Calories; 1.7 g Total Fat (0.9 g Mono, 0.2 g Poly, 0.2 g Sat); 1 mg Cholesterol; 19 g Carbohydrate; 3 g Fibre; 3 g Protein; 110 mg Sodium

CHOICES: 1 Grains & Starches

Pictured on page 90.

Kid-Friendly Idea: Omit green onion, cumin and ginger.

1 serving: 97 Calories; 1.7 g Total Fat (0.9 g Mono, 0.2 g Poly, 0.2 g Sat); 1 mg Cholesterol; 18 g Carbohydrate; 3 g Fibre; 3 g Protein; 110 mg Sodium

CHOICES: 1 Grains & Starches

Spinach Mushroom Rice

The wonderful aroma of jasmine rice is a perfect complement to the spinach and mushroom flavour. Serve with Succulent Lamb Chops, page 37, or Moroccan Chicken, page 64.

Jasmine rice	1 cup	250 mL
Water	1 1/2 cups	375 mL
Canola oil	2 tsp.	10 mL
Finely chopped onion	1 cup	250 mL
Garlic clove, minced	1	1
(or 1/4 tsp., 1 mL, powder)		
Sliced fresh white mushrooms	3 cups	750 mL
Low-sodium prepared chicken broth	1/2 cup	125 mL
Chopped fresh spinach leaves, lightly packed	3 cups	750 mL
Light sour cream	3 tbsp.	50 mL

Combine rice and water in medium saucepan. Bring to a boil. Reduce heat to low. Cover. Cook for 15 minutes. Remove from heat. Let stand for 5 minutes without lifting lid. Fluff with fork. Cover to keep warm.

Heat canola oil in large non-stick frying pan on medium. Add onion and garlic. Cook for about 5 minutes, stirring often, until onion is softened.

Add mushrooms. Cook for 7 to 10 minutes, stirring occasionally, until mushrooms are lightly browned and liquid is evaporated.

Add broth. Bring to a boil. Add spinach. Heat and stir for about 1 minute until spinach is just wilted. Remove from heat.

Stir in sour cream. Add rice. Stir. Makes 4 1/2 cups (1.1 L).

1/2 cup (125 mL): 67 Calories; 1.6 g Total Fat (0.6 g Mono, 0.3 g Poly, 0.3 g Sat); 2 mg Cholesterol; 12 g Carbohydrate; 1 g Fibre; 2 g Protein; 54 mg Sodium

CHOICES: 1/2 Grains & Starches

Pictured on page 53.

Kid-Friendly Idea: Chop spinach and mushrooms quite fine so there are no large pieces.

Creamed Veggie Spaghetti

Lots of colourful vegetables in a creamy, basil-flavoured sauce. Make this dish as spicy as you like by adjusting the fresh chilies, but note it is very spicy as is. Makes a great vegetarian entrée or a side dish for grilled fish or meat.

Whole-wheat spaghetti	8 oz.	225 g
Boiling water	8 cups	2 L
Fresh asparagus, trimmed of tough ends, cut into 2 inch (5 cm) pieces	1 lb.	454 g
Olive oil	1 tbsp.	15 mL
Garlic cloves, minced (or 1/2 tsp., 2 mL, powder)	2	2
Slivered red pepper	1 1/2 cups	375 mL
Sliced fresh brown mushrooms	1 1/2 cups	375 mL
Finely diced fresh red or green chilies (see Tip, page 113)	1 tbsp.	15 mL
Can of skim evaporated milk	13 1/2 oz.	385 mL
Skim milk	1/2 cup	125 mL
Cornstarch	2 tbsp.	30 mL
Finely grated fresh Romano cheese	1/3 cup	75 mL
Finely chopped fresh basil (or 1 1/4 tsp., 6 mL, dried)	1 1/2 tbsp.	25 mL
Pepper	1/2 tsp.	2 mL

Cook spaghetti in boiling water in large uncovered pot or Dutch oven for 6 minutes. Add asparagus. Stir. Boil for 3 to 4 minutes until spaghetti is tender but firm. Drain. Rinse with cold water. Drain well. Transfer to large serving bowl. Cover to keep warm.

Heat olive oil in same large pot on medium. Add next 4 ingredients. Cook for about 5 minutes, stirring often, until vegetables are slightly softened. Add to spaghetti. Cover to keep warm.

Heat evaporated milk in same pot on medium until hot.

Stir skim milk into cornstarch in small cup until smooth. Stir into evaporated milk. Heat and stir until boiling and thickened. Remove from heat.

Add remaining 3 ingredients. Stir until cheese is melted. Add to spaghetti mixture. Toss until coated. Serve immediately. Makes 8 cups (2 L).

(continued on next page)

1 cup (250 mL): 201 Calories; 3.9 g Total Fat (1.3 g Mono, 0.3 g Poly, 1.4 g Sat); 5 mg Cholesterol; 31 g Carbohydrate; 4 g Fibre; 11 g Protein; 155 mg Sodium

CHOICES: 1 Grains & Starches; 1/2 Milk & Alternatives

Pictured on page 108.

Kid-Friendly Idea: Omit fresh chilies and red pepper.

1 cup (250 mL): 197 Calories; 3.8 g Total Fat (1.3 g Mono, 0.3 g Poly, 1.4 g Sat); 5 mg Cholesterol; 30 g Carbohydrate; 4 g Fibre; 11 g Protein; 155 mg Sodium

CHOICES: 1 Grains & Starches; 1/2 Milk & Alternatives

Tomato Herb Pasta

Rich flavour in a light tomato and herb sauce. Even better with a sprinkle of fresh Parmesan or ricotta cheese.

Boiling water	9 cups	2.25 L
Salt	1/4 tsp.	1 mL
Penne pasta	3 cups	750 mL
Olive (or canola) oil	2 tsp.	10 mL
Finely chopped red onion	1 cup	250 mL
Garlic clove, minced (or 1/4 tsp., 1 mL, powder)	1	1
Medium Roma (plum) tomatoes, chopped	6	6
Chopped fresh basil (or 1 1/2 tsp., 7 mL, dried)	2 tbsp.	30 mL
Chopped fresh parsley (or 1 1/2 tsp., 7 mL, flakes)	2 tbsp.	30 mL
Sweet chili sauce	1 – 2 tbsp.	15 – 30 mL

Combine boiling water and salt in large pot or Dutch oven. Add pasta. Cook, uncovered, for 12 to 15 minutes, stirring occasionally, until tender but firm. Drain well. Return to pot. Cover to keep warm.

Heat olive oil in large frying pan on medium. Add onion and garlic. Cook for 5 to 10 minutes, stirring often, until onion is softened.

Add remaining 4 ingredients. Heat and stir for about 5 minutes until tomatoes are softened. Add to pasta. Toss. Makes 5 cups (1.25 L).

1 cup (250 mL): 306 Calories; 3.3 g Total Fat (1.4 g Mono, 0.4 g Poly, 0.3 g Sat); 0 mg Cholesterol; 59 g Carbohydrate; 4 g Fibre; 10 g Protein; 35 mg Sodium

CHOICES: 3 Grains & Starches; 1 Vegetables

Creamy Corn and Onion

Caramelized onion and parsley add extra flavour to sweet corn.

Canola oil	2 tsp.	10 mL
Thinly sliced onion	1 cup	250 mL
All-purpose flour	2 tsp.	10 mL
Brown sugar, packed	1 tsp.	5 mL
Balsamic vinegar	1 tsp.	5 mL
Salt, sprinkle		
Milk	3/4 cup	175 mL
Pepper	1/4 tsp.	1 mL
Can of kernel corn, drained	12 oz.	341 mL
Chopped fresh parsley	3 tbsp.	50 mL
(or 2 1/4 tsp., 11 mL, flakes)		

Heat canola oil in large frying pan on medium. Add onion. Cook for about 10 minutes, stirring often, until onion is soft and golden.

Add next 4 ingredients. Heat and stir for 1 minute.

Stir in milk. Add pepper. Heat and stir for about 2 minutes until boiling and thickened.

Add corn and parsley. Heat and stir until corn is heated through. Makes about 2 cups (500 mL).

1/2 cup (125 mL): 141 Calories; 2.9 g Total Fat (1.5 g Mono, 0.7 g Poly, 0.5 g Sat); 3 mg Cholesterol; 24 g Carbohydrate; 3 g Fibre; 4 g Protein; 282 mg Sodium

CHOICES: 1 Grains & Starches; 1/2 Fats

Paré Pointer

Bread is actually raw toast.

Side Dishes

Crunchy Rice Salad

Bright, crispy vegetables with rice and pineapple. Coconut gives the salad unique flavour.

Cold cooked jasmine rice (2/3 cup, 150 mL, uncooked)	2 cups	500 mL
Can of pineapple tidbits, drained	14 oz.	398 mL
Can of water chestnuts, drained and chopped	8 oz.	227 mL
Diced celery	1/2 cup	125 mL
Diced red pepper	1/2 cup	125 mL
Diced red onion	1/2 cup	125 mL
LIME DRESSING		
Lime juice	3 tbsp.	50 mL
Canola oil	1 tbsp.	15 mL
Low-sodium soy sauce	1 tbsp.	15 mL
Sweet chili sauce	1 tbsp.	15 mL
Long thread coconut, toasted (see Tip, below)	1/4 cup	60 mL

Toss first 6 ingredients in large bowl.

Lime Dressing: Combine first 4 ingredients in jar with tight-fitting lid. Shake well. Makes 1/3 cup (75 mL) dressing. Drizzle over rice mixture. Toss. Sprinkle with coconut. Makes 5 cups (1.25 L).

1/2 cup (125 mL): 85 Calories; 2.7 g Total Fat (0.9 g Mono, 0.4 g Poly, 1.2 g Sat); 0 mg Cholesterol; 16 g Carbohydrate; 2 g Fibre; 1 g Protein; 80 mg Sodium

CHOICES: 1/2 Fruits

Pictured on page 108.

 When toasting nuts, seeds or coconut, cooking times will vary for each type of nut—so never toast them together. For small amounts, place ingredient in an ungreased frying pan. Heat on medium for 3 to 5 minutes, stirring often, until golden. For larger amounts, spread ingredient evenly in an ungreased shallow pan. Bake in a 350°F (175°C) oven for 5 to 10 minutes, stirring or shaking often, until golden.

Fried Rice

Very colourful with peas, green onion and red pepper. Earthy Chinese
mushroom flavour with a nice crunch from fresh bean sprouts.

Chinese dried mushrooms	6	6
Boiling water	2 cups	500 mL
Canola oil	2 tsp.	10 mL
Chopped green onion	1/3 cup	75 mL
Finely chopped red pepper	1/2 cup	125 mL
Cooked long grain white rice (1 cup, 250 mL, uncooked)	3 cups	750 mL
Frozen peas	1/2 cup	125 mL
Finely chopped fat-free cooked ham	1/3 cup	75 mL
Low-sodium soy sauce	2 tbsp.	30 mL
Chili powder	1/2 tsp.	2 mL
Fresh bean sprouts, trimmed	1 1/2 cups	375 mL

Put mushrooms into small bowl. Cover with boiling water. Let stand for about 20 minutes until softened. Drain. Remove and discard stems. Finely chop caps.

Heat wok or large frying pan on medium until hot. Add canola oil. Add green onion and red pepper. Stir-fry for about 1 minute until onion is softened.

Add mushrooms. Add next 5 ingredients. Stir-fry for about 5 minutes until hot.

Add bean sprouts. Stir-fry about 1 minute until heated through. Makes 6 cups (1.5 L).

1 cup (250 mL): 182 Calories; 2.4 g Total Fat (1.0 g Mono, 0.6 g Poly, 0.3 g Sat); 4 mg Cholesterol; 33 g Carbohydrate; 3 g Fibre; 8 g Protein; 367 mg Sodium

CHOICES: 1 1/2 Grains & Starches; 1 Vegetables

Pictured on page 17.

Kid-Friendly Idea: Omit the mushrooms and bean sprouts.

1 cup (250 mL): 150 Calories; 2.3 g Total Fat (1.0 g Mono, 0.5 g Poly, 0.3 g Sat); 4 mg Cholesterol; 26 g Carbohydrate; 1 g Fibre; 6 g Protein; 365 mg Sodium

CHOICES: 1 1/2 Grains & Starches

Mushroom Polenta

Peppery mushroom flavours in a thick, creamy textured polenta. An attractive alternative to pasta or potato.

Canola oil	2 tsp.	10 mL
Sliced fresh white mushrooms	2 cups	500 mL
Salt	1/4 tsp.	1 mL
Low-sodium prepared chicken broth	4 cups	1 L
Yellow cornmeal	1 1/2 cups	375 mL
Grated low-fat medium Cheddar cheese	1/2 cup	125 mL
Chopped fresh chives	3 tbsp.	50 mL
(or 2 1/2 tsp., 12 mL, dried)		
Pepper	1/4 tsp.	1 mL

Heat canola oil in large saucepan on medium-high. Add mushrooms and salt. Heat and stir for about 5 minutes until mushrooms are softened and beginning to brown. Transfer to small bowl.

Heat broth in same saucepan until boiling. Reduce heat to medium-low. Add cornmeal in slow, steady stream, stirring constantly. Heat and stir for about 10 minutes until soft and thick.

Add mushrooms. Add remaining 3 ingredients. Stir. Spread cornmeal mixture evenly in greased 9 x 13 inch (23 x 33 cm) pan. Cool for 30 minutes. Cover. Chill for 1 to 2 hours until set. Cut into 12 equal pieces. Spray both sides of polenta pieces with cooking spray. Cook in large greased frying pan or on greased electric grill or gas barbecue on medium for about 3 minutes per side until lightly golden. Makes 12 pieces.

1 piece: 92 Calories; 2.8 g Total Fat (1.0 g Mono, 0.4 g Poly, 1.3 g Sat); 7 mg Cholesterol; 13 g Carbohydrate; 1 g Fibre; 4 g Protein; 338 mg Sodium

CHOICES: 1 Grains & Starches

Pictured on page 71.

Crispy Spiced Potatoes

Flavourful herb and spice-speckled potato wedges. Outside edges are crispy and inside is soft and moist.

Egg whites (large), room temperature	2	2
Large red potatoes	4	4
Chopped fresh rosemary	2 tsp.	10 mL
Lemon pepper	1 tsp.	5 mL
Ground cumin	1/2 tsp.	2 mL
Garlic powder	1/2 tsp.	2 mL

Beat egg whites in extra-large bowl until just frothy. Do not overbeat.

Cut potatoes in half lengthwise. Cut each half lengthwise into 4 wedges. Add to egg whites. Toss until coated. Arrange in single layer on greased baking sheet.

Combine remaining 4 ingredients in small bowl. Sprinkle over potato wedges. Bake in 400°F (205°C) oven for about 1 hour, turning after 30 minutes, until crisp and golden. Makes 32 wedges.

4 wedges: 87 Calories; 0.2 g Total Fat (trace Mono, 0.1 g Poly, trace Sat); 0 mg Cholesterol; 18 g Carbohydrate; 2 g Fibre; 3 g Protein; 36 mg Sodium

CHOICES: 1 Grains & Starches

Pictured on front cover and on page 89.

Kid-Friendly Idea: Take away their forks and add a small bowl of light sour cream or ketchup for dipping. Kids will usually eat potatoes this way.

Paré Pointer
A Scotland Yard has three feet just like anywhere else.

Side Dishes

Potato Salad

A wonderful mix of red potatoes and crisp radishes in a creamy yogurt dressing. The goat cheese adds a zesty burst of flavour.

Baby red potatoes, halved	2 lbs.	900 g
Water		
Ice water		
Thinly sliced radishes	3/4 cup	175 mL
Alfalfa sprouts	2/3 cup	150 mL
Soft goat (chevré) cheese	3 oz.	85 g
YOGURT AND HERB DRESSING		
Low-fat plain yogurt	1/2 cup	125 mL
Low-fat French dressing	2 tbsp.	30 mL
Chopped fresh mint leaves	2 tbsp.	30 mL
(or 1 1/2 tsp., 7 mL, dried)		
Chopped fresh chives	2 tbsp.	30 mL
(or 1 1/2 tsp., 7 mL, dried)		

Cook potato in water in large pot or Dutch oven on medium for about 15 minutes until just tender. Drain. Immediately plunge potato into large bowl of ice water. Let stand for about 5 minutes until cool. Drain well. Remove to paper towels to dry completely. Transfer to separate large bowl.

Add next 3 ingredients. Stir.

Yogurt and Herb Dressing: Combine all 4 ingredients in jar with tight-fitting lid. Shake well. Makes 2/3 cup (150 mL) dressing. Drizzle over potato mixture. Toss. Makes 6 cups (1.5 L).

1 cup (250 mL): 203 Calories; 3.5 g Total Fat (0.7 g Mono, 0.1 g Poly, 2.4 g Sat); 9 mg Cholesterol; 33 g Carbohydrate; 2 g Fibre; 9 g Protein; 145 mg Sodium

CHOICES: 2 Grains & Starches

Pictured on page 108.

Kid-Friendly Idea: Omit the radishes, alfalfa sprouts and goat cheese. Add 1/2 cup (125 mL) grated light sharp Cheddar cheese. Omit mint leaves and chives in dressing.

1 cup (250 mL): 185 Calories; 2.0 g Total Fat (trace Mono, 0 g Poly, 1.3 g Sat); 8 mg Cholesterol; 33 g Carbohydrate; 2 g Fibre; 9 g Protein; 143 mg Sodium

CHOICES: 1 1/2 Grains & Starches; 1/2 Milk & Alternatives; 1/2 Meat & Alternatives

Potato and Fennel Bake

Fennel and potatoes baked with fresh dill and Parmesan cheese. A unique and elegant way to serve potatoes with the Sunday roast.

Large peeled potatoes, cut crosswise into 1/4 inch (6 mm) slices	3	3
Large fennel bulb (white part only), thinly sliced	1	1
Chopped fresh dill (or 1 1/4 tsp., 6 mL, dried)	1 1/2 tbsp.	25 mL
Low-sodium prepared chicken broth	1/2 cup	125 mL
Milk	1/2 cup	125 mL
Finely grated fresh Parmesan cheese	3 tbsp.	50 mL
Chopped fresh dill (or 1 1/4 tsp., 6 mL, dried)	1 1/2 tbsp.	25 mL
Pepper	1/2 tsp.	2 mL

Arrange half of potato in lightly greased shallow 3 quart (3 L) casserole. Arrange half of fennel over potato.

Sprinkle with first amount of dill. Layer with remaining potatoes and fennel.

Combine broth and milk in 1 cup (250 mL) liquid measure. Pour over potato mixture.

Sprinkle with remaining 3 ingredients. Cover. Bake in 350°F (175°C) oven for 30 minutes. Remove cover. Bake, uncovered, for about 30 minutes until potato is tender and top is browned. Serves 8.

1 serving: 91 Calories; 1.0 g Total Fat (0.1 g Mono, 0 g Poly, 0.5 g Sat); 3 mg Cholesterol; 19 g Carbohydrate; 3 g Fibre; 5 g Protein; 108 mg Sodium

CHOICES: 1 Grains & Starches

Roasted Cauliflower

A tasty way to cook cauliflower. Roasting brings out a wonderful earthy flavour.

Cauliflower florets	6 cups	1.5 L
Canola oil	1 1/2 tbsp.	25 mL
Ground nutmeg	1/2 tsp.	2 mL
Garlic powder	1/4 tsp.	1 mL
Pepper	1/4 tsp.	1 mL

Toss all 5 ingredients in large bowl. Spread on greased baking sheet. Bake in 375°F (190°C) oven for about 30 minutes until cauliflower is tender-crisp. Makes 4 cups (1 L).

1 cup (250 mL): 85 Calories; 5.5 g Total Fat (3.0 g Mono, 1.6 g Poly, 0.5 g Sat); 0 mg Cholesterol; 8 g Carbohydrate; 4 g Fibre; 3 g Protein; 45 mg Sodium

CHOICES: 1 Vegetables; 1 Fats

Pictured on page 125.

Mashed Sweet Potatoes

This smooth, creamy purée has flecks of green parsley.

Canola oil	2 tsp.	10 mL
Thinly sliced onion	1 cup	250 mL
Water		
Salt	1/4 tsp.	1 mL
Chopped peeled orange-fleshed sweet potato	4 cups	1 L
Low-fat plain yogurt	2 – 3 tbsp.	30 – 50 mL
Chopped fresh parsley (or 3/4 – 1 1/2 tsp., 4 – 7 mL, flakes)	1 – 2 tbsp.	15 – 30 mL

Heat canola oil in medium frying pan on medium. Add onion. Cook for about 15 minutes, stirring often, until onion is softened.

Combine water and salt in medium saucepan on medium-high. Add sweet potato. Cook for about 15 minutes until tender. Drain well. Return to saucepan. Mash until no lumps remain.

Add yogurt, parsley and onion mixture. Stir well. Makes 2 1/2 cups (625 mL).

1/2 cup (125 mL): 121 Calories; 2.0 g Total Fat (1.1 g Mono, 0.6 g Poly, 0.2 g Sat); 0.4 mg Cholesterol; 24 g Carbohydrate; 4 g Fibre; 2 g Protein; 122 mg Sodium

CHOICES: 1 Grains & Starches

Side Dishes

Maple Butternut Squash

A comforting, colourful side dish that is great served with stew or even warm in a fresh green salad. Peppery and vibrant, with a hint of rosemary.

Cubed butternut squash	5 cups	1.25 L
Canola oil	2 tsp.	10 mL
Garlic cloves, bruised (see Note)	2	2
Sprigs of fresh rosemary	2	2
Salt	1/4 tsp.	1 mL
Pepper	1/4 tsp.	1 mL
Maple syrup	1 tbsp.	15 mL

Put first 6 ingredients into large bowl. Toss until evenly coated. Transfer to greased baking sheet. Bake, uncovered, in 400°F (205°C) oven for about 40 minutes, stirring once, until edges start to turn brown. Discard rosemary sprigs.

Drizzle with maple syrup. Toss. Bake for about 10 minutes until glazed and golden. Makes 2 cups (500 mL).

1/2 cup (125 mL): 171 Calories; 2.7 g Total Fat (1.4 g Mono, 0.8 g Poly, 0.2 g Sat); 0 mg Cholesterol; 39 g Carbohydrate; 6 g Fibre; 3 g Protein; 158 mg Sodium

CHOICES: 6 Vegetables; 1/2 Fats

Pictured on page 125.

Note: To bruise garlic cloves, hit cloves with a mallet or the flat side of a wide knife to "bruise" or crush them slightly.

Kid-Friendly Idea: Omit garlic cloves and rosemary.

Paré Pointer
At night, the prettiest fish are starfish

Zucchini Pepper Combo

Simplicity in seasoning and cooking brings out the best flavour of these tender-crisp, perfectly cooked vegetables. All the "juices" form a tasty sauce.

Medium zucchini (with peel), quartered lengthwise, seeded	2	2
Olive oil	2 tsp.	10 mL
Red medium pepper, diced	1	1
Yellow or orange medium pepper, diced	1	1
Lemon pepper	1/2 tsp.	2 mL
Balsamic vinegar	2 tsp.	10 mL
Pepper	1/4 tsp.	1 mL

Cut zucchini crosswise into 1/2 inch (12 mm) pieces.

Heat olive oil in large non-stick frying pan or wok on medium-high. Add zucchini, red and yellow peppers and lemon pepper. Stir-fry for 5 to 7 minutes until tender-crisp.

Sprinkle with balsamic vinegar and pepper. Stir. Serve immediately. Makes 3 cups (750 mL).

1/2 cup (125 mL): 26 Calories; 1.7 g Total Fat (0.9 g Mono, 0.5 g Poly, 0.1 g Sat); 0 mg Cholesterol; 3 g Carbohydrate; 1 g Fibre; trace Protein; 11 mg Sodium

CHOICES: No Choices

Pictured on page 18.

Kid-Friendly Idea: Omit the balsamic vinegar and sprinkle of pepper. Substitute with 2 tsp. (10 mL) low-fat Italian dressing.

1/2 cup (125 mL): 25 Calories; 1.7 g Total Fat (0.9 g Mono, 0.5 g Poly, 0.1 g Sat); trace Cholesterol; 3 g Carbohydrate; 1 g Fibre; 1 g Protein; 18 mg Sodium

CHOICES: No Choices

Creamy Spinach

Fast and easy with lots of flavour. Goes well with grilled chicken or beef.

Hard margarine (or butter)	2 tsp.	10 mL
Finely chopped onion	1 cup	250 mL
Garlic clove, minced (or 1/4 tsp., 1 mL, powder)	1	1
Fresh spinach leaves, lightly packed	6 cups	1.5 L
Ground nutmeg	1/4 tsp.	1 mL
Lemon pepper	1/4 tsp.	1 mL
Light sour cream	2 tbsp.	30 mL

Melt margarine in large frying pan on medium. Add onion and garlic. Cook for 5 to 10 minutes, stirring often, until onion is softened.

Add spinach. Heat and stir for about 3 minutes until spinach is almost wilted.

Add remaining 3 ingredients. Heat and stir until combined. Makes about 1 1/2 cups (375 mL).

1/2 cup (125 mL): 75 Calories; 3.7 g Total Fat (1.5 g Mono, 0.7 g Poly, 1.0 g Sat); 3 mg Cholesterol; 9 g Carbohydrate; 2 g Fibre; 3 g Protein; 110 mg Sodium

CHOICES: 1 Vegetables; 1/2 Fats

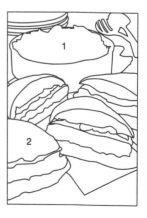

1. Spinach and Pork Salad, page 87
2. Grilled Pork Sandwiches, page 86

Props courtesy of: Cherison Enterprises Inc.

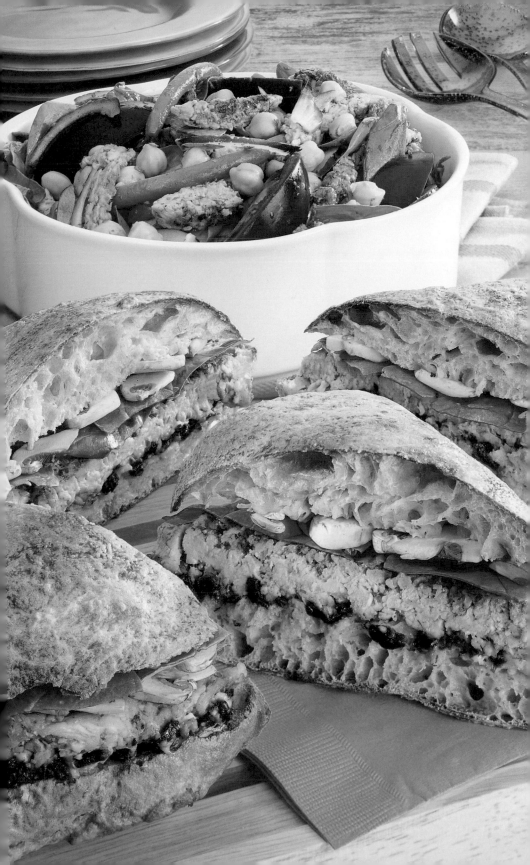

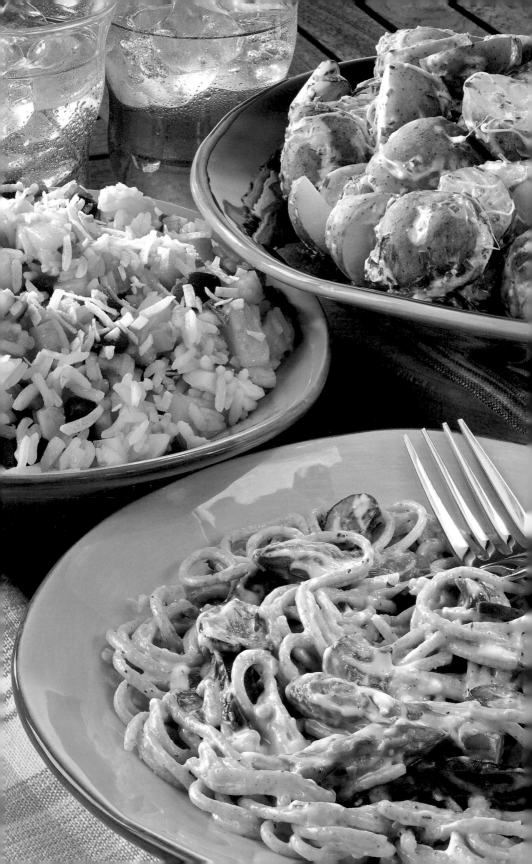

Asparagus and Mushrooms

Tender-crisp, green asparagus is tasty with a fresh lemon flavour and honey sweetness. An elegant presentation.

Hard margarine (or butter)	2 tsp.	10 mL
Sliced fresh white mushrooms	2 cups	500 mL
Fresh asparagus, trimmed of tough ends	1 lb.	454 g
Chopped fresh parsley (or 2 1/4 tsp., 11 mL, flakes)	3 tbsp.	50 mL
Liquid honey	2 tsp.	10 mL
Finely grated lemon zest	1/4 tsp.	1 mL
Salt	1/4 tsp.	1 mL

Melt margarine in large frying pan on medium-high. Add mushrooms and asparagus. Heat for about 5 minutes, stirring occasionally, until asparagus is tender-crisp.

Add remaining 4 ingredients. Heat and stir for about 30 seconds until combined. Serves 4.

1 serving: 60 Calories; 2.1 g Total Fat (1.1 g Mono, 0.5 g Poly, 0.4 g Sat); 0 mg Cholesterol; 9 g Carbohydrate; 2 g Fibre; 3 g Protein; 174 mg Sodium

CHOICES: No Choices

Pictured on front cover and on page 36.

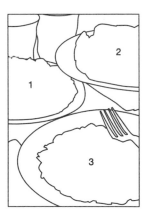

1. Crunchy Rice Salad, page 97
2. Potato Salad, page 101
3. Creamed Veggie Spaghetti, page 94

Props courtesy of: Danesco Inc.

Pea Medley

Sweet, tender-crisp peas glazed with butter. The fresh mint flavour goes delightfully well with the peas.

Low-sodium prepared chicken broth	2 tbsp.	30 mL
Green onions, cut into 1 inch (2.5 cm) pieces	8	8
Garlic clove, minced (or 1/4 tsp., 1 mL, powder)	1	1
Sugar snap peas	2 cups	500 mL
Fresh snow peas	2 cups	500 mL
Frozen peas	1 cup	250 mL
Salt	1/4 tsp.	1 mL
Pepper	1/4 tsp.	1 mL
Chopped fresh mint	2 tbsp.	30 mL
Hard margarine (or butter)	2 tsp.	10 mL

Heat broth in non-stick wok or large frying pan on medium-high. Add green onion and garlic. Stir-fry for about 1 minute until fragrant.

Add next 5 ingredients. Cook, uncovered, for 2 to 3 minutes, stirring often, until peas are tender-crisp. Do not overcook.

Add mint and margarine. Stir-fry for about 30 seconds until margarine is melted and peas are coated. Serve immediately. Makes 4 cups (1 L).

2/3 cup (150 mL): 76 Calories; 1.4 g Total Fat (0.7 g Mono, 0.3 g Poly, 0.3 g Sat); trace Cholesterol; 12 g Carbohydrate; 4 g Fibre; 4 g Protein; 151 mg Sodium

CHOICES: 2 Vegetables

Pictured on page 125.

Kid-Friendly Idea: Omit garlic and mint.

Oven-Fried Vegetables

Enjoy these for the taste of deep-fried vegetables without the fat. These crisp mixed vegetables are lightly breaded and baked. Serve with Spicy Roasted Pepper Sauce, page 113, as a dip.

Low-cholesterol egg product (see Note 1, below)	1/2 cup	125 mL
Blanched mixed vegetable pieces (see Note 2, below)	2 lbs.	900 g
Fine cornflake crumbs	1 cup	250 mL
Garlic and herb no-salt seasoning	1 1/2 tsp.	7 mL

Put egg product into large bowl. Add vegetables. Stir until coated.

Combine crumbs and seasoning in large resealable freezer bag. Add vegetables, in small batches. Shake until coated. Arrange in single layer on greased baking sheet. Spray vegetables well with cooking spray. Bake in 400°F (205°C) oven for about 20 minutes until browned. Makes about 6 cups (1.5 L). Serves 6.

1 serving: 125 Calories; 1.8 g Total Fat (0.4 g Mono, 1.0 g Poly, 0.3 g Sat); trace Cholesterol; 21 g Carbohydrate; 4 g Fibre; 6 g Protein; 194 mq Sodium

CHOICES: 1 Vegetables; 1 Grains & Starches

Pictured on page 125.

Note 1: 3 tbsp. (50 mL) egg product is equivalent to 1 large egg. Recipe needs 1/2 cup (125 mL) egg product to coat vegetables, however, about 2 tbsp. (30 mL) will be discarded from bottom of bowl after coating.

Note 2: Blanch broccoli and cauliflower florets, bell pepper pieces and zucchini spears in boiling water for 1 minute and then plunge into ice water. Partially cook hard vegetables (such as halved baby potatoes, peeled winter squash and turnip chunks, and carrot and parsnip pieces) by boiling or steaming for 3 to 5 minutes until just barely tender, and then plunging into ice water.

Onion and Garlic Dipping Sauce

The perfect sauce for dipping vegetables. Makes a great topping for a baked potato as well. Excellent with Blackened Snapper, page 23.

Light sour cream	2/3 cup	150 mL
Non-fat mayonnaise	1/3 cup	75 mL
Garlic cloves	3	3
Lemon juice	2 tbsp.	30 mL
Olive oil	1 tbsp.	15 mL
Finely grated lemon zest	1/4 tsp.	1 mL
Green onions, finely chopped	2	2

Process first 6 ingredients in blender or food processor, scraping down sides as necessary, until smooth. Pour into small bowl.

Stir in green onion. Cover. Chill for 30 minutes to blend flavours. Makes 1 cup (250 mL).

2 tbsp. (30 mL): 60 Calories; 4.6 g Total Fat (1.2 g Mono, 0.3 g Poly, 1.5 g Sat); 6 mg Cholesterol; 4 g Carbohydrate; trace Fibre; 1 g Protein; 126 mg Sodium

CHOICES: 1 Fats

Lightened-Up Cheese Sauce

This creamy sauce has a sharp cheese flavour. Great on steamed vegetables, potatoes or an egg white omelet.

Skim milk	1 1/4 cups	300 mL
All-purpose flour	3 tbsp.	50 mL
Grated light sharp Cheddar cheese	1 1/2 cups	375 mL
Non-fat garlic-herb cream cheese	1/4 cup	60 mL
Seasoned salt	1/2 tsp.	2 mL
Dry mustard	1/4 tsp.	1 mL
Paprika	1/4 tsp.	1 mL

Stir milk into flour in medium saucepan until smooth. Heat and stir on medium until boiling and thickened. Reduce heat to low.

(continued on next page)

Add remaining 5 ingredients. Heat and stir until both cheeses are melted. Makes 2 cups (500 mL).

1/4 cup (60 mL):): 82 Calories; 3.4 g Total Fat (0 g Mono, trace Poly, 2.3 g Sat); 13 mg Cholesterol; 5 g Carbohydrate; trace Fibre; 9 g Protein; 285 mg Sodium

CHOICES: 1 Meat & Alternatives

Spicy Roasted Pepper Sauce

A thick sauce with a hint of jalapeño. Serve with chicken, beef or lamb, or toss through pasta. Can also be used as a pizza sauce or dip. If you prefer a hotter sauce, leave the seeds in the jalapeño pepper.

Red medium peppers, quartered	6	6
Medium onions, cut lengthwise into wedges	2	2
Garlic cloves	2	2
Medium jalapeño pepper, seeds and ribs removed (see Tip, below)	1	1
Olive (or canola) oil	1 tbsp.	15 mL
Brown sugar, packed	1 tsp.	5 mL
Salt	1/4 tsp.	1 mL
Pepper	1/4 tsp.	1 mL

Combine all 8 ingredients on greased large baking sheet. Bake in 375°F (190°C) oven for about 1 hour, stirring occasionally, until pepper and onion are soft and browned. Cool. Process in blender or food processor until smooth. Makes about 3 cups (750 mL).

1/4 cup (60 mL): 38 Calories; 1.4 g Total Fat (0.8 g Mono, 0.3 g Poly, 0.2 g Sat); 0 mg Cholesterol; 7 g Carbohydrate; 2 g Fibre; 1 g Protein; 51 mg Sodium

CHOICES: 1 Vegetables

Pictured on page 36.

Kid-Friendly Idea: Omit the jalapeño pepper.

 tip Wear rubber gloves when cutting jalapeño peppers and avoid touching your eyes.

Creamy Mushroom Sauce

A creamy, golden-brown sauce that mushroom lovers will adore! Perfect over steak or chicken.

Canola oil	1 tbsp.	15 mL
Sliced fresh brown mushrooms	2 cups	500 mL
Hard margarine (or butter)	1 tbsp.	15 mL
Garlic clove, minced	1	1
(or 1/4 tsp., 1 mL, powder)		
All-purpose flour	1 tbsp.	15 mL
Low-sodium prepared chicken broth	1 cup	250 mL
Dry (or alcohol-free) white wine	1/2 cup	125 mL
Light sour cream	2 tbsp.	30 mL
Chopped fresh chives	2 tbsp.	30 mL
(or 1 1/2 tsp., 7 mL, dried)		
Salt	1/4 tsp.	1 mL
Pepper	1/4 tsp.	1 mL

Heat canola oil in large frying pan on medium. Add mushrooms. Cook for about 5 minutes, stirring occasionally, until lightly browned. Remove to small bowl.

Add margarine and garlic to same frying pan. Heat and stir on medium for about 1 minute until garlic is fragrant. Add flour. Heat and stir for 1 minute.

Add mushrooms, broth and wine. Cook and stir for about 5 minutes until boiling and thickened.

Add remaining 4 ingredients. Heat and stir for about 2 minutes until well combined. Makes about 1 1/4 cups (300 mL).

2 tbsp. (30 mL): 44 Calories; 2.9 g Total Fat (1.5 g Mono, 0.7 g Poly, 0.5 g Sat); 2 mg Cholesterol; 2 g Carbohydrate; trace Fibre; 1 g Protein; 93 mg Sodium

CHOICES: 1/2 Fats

Tropical Yogurt Topping

This creamy topping has a wonderful banana flavour. Delicious on burgers or sandwiches.

Plain yogurt, drained (see Note)	3/4 cup	175 mL
Brown sugar, packed	1 tbsp.	15 mL
Dark rum	1 tbsp.	15 mL
Lemon juice	2 tsp.	10 mL
Salt	1/4 tsp.	1 mL
Can of pineapple slices, drained, diced	14 oz.	398 mL
Chopped fresh parsley (or 2 1/4 tsp., 11 mL, flakes)	3 tbsp.	50 mL
Medium bananas, diced	2	2

Combine first 5 ingredients in medium bowl. Stir until sugar is dissolved.

Add pineapple and parsley. Stir.

Gently fold in banana until coated. Makes 2 1/4 cups (550 mL).

1/4 cup (60 mL): 72 Calories; 0.1 g Total Fat (trace Mono, trace Poly, trace Sat); 0.6 mg Cholesterol; 16 g Carbohydrate; 1 g Fibre; 2 g Protein; 86 mg Sodium

CHOICES: 1 Fruits

Variation: Omit chopped fresh parsley. Use same amount of finely chopped fresh mint.

Paré Pointer

Chickens keep in shape by eggs-ercising.

Apple Cranberry Chutney

This chutney is great with pork or roasted turkey. Make ahead of time and freeze in an airtight container.

Chopped, peeled tart cooking apples (such as Granny Smith)	5 cups	1.25 L
Dried cranberries	1 cup	250 mL
White wine vinegar	1/2 cup	125 mL
Apple juice	1/2 cup	125 mL
Brown sugar, packed	1/4 cup	60 mL
Cinnamon stick (4 inches, 10 cm)	1	1
Ground ginger	1/2 tsp.	2 mL
Ground cloves	1/16 tsp.	0.5 mL
Salt	1/4 tsp.	1 mL

Combine all 9 ingredients in large pot or Dutch oven. Heat and stir on medium until sugar is dissolved. Bring to a boil. Reduce heat to medium-low. Simmer, uncovered, for about 40 minutes, stirring occasionally, until thickened and most of liquid is evaporated. Remove and discard cinnamon stick. Makes about 3 1/4 cups (800 mL).

2 tbsp. (30 mL): 36 Calories; 0.1 g Total Fat (0 g Mono, trace Poly, trace Sat); 0 mg Cholesterol; 10 g Carbohydrate; 1 g Fibre; trace Protein; 23 mg Sodium

CHOICES: 1/2 Fruits

Pictured on page 53.

Apricot Clafouti

Pronounced kla-FOO-tee. A custard-like dessert that is equally as good with cherries, plums or peaches in place of apricots. Sprinkle top with sliced almonds for a subtle nutty flavour and texture.

All-purpose flour	1/2 cup	125 mL
Whole-wheat flour	2 tbsp.	30 mL
Granulated sugar	1/3 cup	75 mL
Buttermilk	1 3/4 cups	425 mL
Low-cholesterol egg product (see Note)	1 cup	250 mL
Ground nutmeg	1/2 tsp.	2 mL
Can of apricot halves, drained	14 oz.	398 mL

Combine both flours and sugar in large bowl.

Combine next 3 ingredients in medium bowl. Pour over flour mixture. Whisk until smooth.

Cut each apricot piece in half. Arrange apricots in bottom of greased 9 inch (23 cm) pie plate. Carefully pour batter over apricots. Bake in 350°F (175°C) oven for 40 to 45 minutes until set. Serve warm or at room temperature. Serves 6.

1 serving: 209 Calories; 5 g Total Fat (1 g Mono, 2.5 g Poly, 1 g Sat); 6 mg Cholesterol; 33 g Carbohydrate; 2 g Fibre; 9 g Protein; 119 mg Sodium

CHOICES: 1/2 Grains & Starches; 1/2 Fruits; 1/2 Meat & Alternatives; 1 Other Choices

Note: 3 tbsp. (50 mL) frozen egg product, thawed, is equivalent to 1 large egg.

Blueberry Cobbler

A warm, comforting, old-fashioned dessert. Serve with low-fat ice cream, frozen yogurt or low-fat custard for a special treat.

Hard margarine (or butter), melted	1/4 cup	60 mL
All-purpose flour	1 cup	250 mL
Milk	3/4 cup	175 mL
Granulated sugar	2 tbsp.	30 mL
Baking powder	2 tsp.	10 mL
Vanilla	1 tsp.	5 mL
Ground cinnamon	1/2 tsp.	2 mL
Ground nutmeg	1/4 tsp.	1 mL
Fresh (or frozen, thawed) blueberries	2 cups	500 mL
Granulated sugar	2 tbsp.	30 mL
Finely grated lemon zest	1 tsp.	5 mL
Water	1/2 cup	125 mL

Pour margarine into bottom of lightly greased 1 1/2 quart (1.5 L) casserole.

Combine next 7 ingredients in medium bowl. Dollop evenly over margarine.

Combine next 3 ingredients in medium bowl. Sprinkle over flour mixture.

Drizzle with water. Do not stir. Bake, uncovered, in 350°F (175°C) oven for 40 to 45 minutes until bubbling and lightly browned. Serves 6.

1 serving: 222 Calories; 8.1 g Total Fat (4.5 g Mono, 1.8 g Poly, 1.5 g Sat); 2 mg Cholesterol; 35 g Carbohydrate; 2 g Fibre; 4 g Protein; 655 mg Sodium

CHOICES: 1 Grains & Starches; 1/2 Fruits; 1/2 Other Choices; 1 1/2 Fats

Strawberry Shortcakes

Deliciously light and airy tea biscuits topped with strawberry
(or your favourite) jam.

BUTTERMILK TEA BISCUITS

All-purpose flour	1 1/2 cups	375 mL
Baking powder	2 tsp.	10 mL
Salt, just a pinch		
Hard margarine (or butter)	2 tbsp.	30 mL
Buttermilk	3/4 cup	175 mL
Salt	1/8 tsp.	0.5 mL
Sugar-free strawberry jam	1/3 cup	75 mL
Low-fat plain yogurt	1/3 cup	75 mL
Fresh strawberries, quartered (for garnish)	2	2

Buttermilk Tea Biscuits: Combine first 3 ingredients in medium bowl. Cut in margarine until mixture resembles coarse crumbs.

Add buttermilk and second amount of salt. Stir until just moistened. Do not overmix. Let stand for 10 minutes. Lightly press out dough on lightly floured surface to 1 inch (2.5 cm) thickness. Cut out circles from dough using lightly floured 2 inch (5 cm) cookie cutter. Arrange circles in single layer, almost touching, in lightly greased 9 x 9 inch (23 x 23 cm) pan. Bake in 450°F (230°C) oven for 10 to 12 minutes until well risen and lightly browned on top and bottom. Let stand in pan for 5 minutes before removing to wire rack to cool. Makes 8 biscuits.

Carefully split each biscuit in half. Place 2 halves, cut side up, on each of 8 dessert plates. Spread each side with jam. Top with small dollop of yogurt and strawberry quarter. Makes 16 biscuit halves. Serves 8.

1 serving: 126 Calories; 3.1 g Total Fat (1.7 g Mono, 0.7 g Poly, 0.6 g Sat); 2 mg Cholesterol; 23 g Carbohydrate; trace Fibre; 4 g Protein; 227 mg Sodium

CHOICES: 1 Grains & Starches; 1/2 Fats

Pictured on page 126.

Tropical Trifles

Kids and adults alike will love these attractive parfaits. A wonderful combination of colours, flavours and textures.

Package of sugar-free lime-flavoured jelly powder	1/3 oz.	10.3 g
Vanilla wafers, coarsely crushed	12	12
Can of pineapple tidbits, drained	14 oz.	398 mL
Low-fat tropical fruit yogurt	1 cup	250 mL
Toasted sliced almonds (see Tip, page 97)	2 tbsp.	30 mL

Prepare jelly powder according to package directions. Pour into 9 x 9 inch (23 x 23 cm) pan. Chill until set. Cut into cubes.

Spoon crushed wafers into six 9 oz. (255 mL) serving glasses. Top with pineapple, jelly and yogurt.

Sprinkle tops with almonds. Serves 6.

1 serving: 145 Calories; 3.2 g Total Fat (0.9 g Mono, 0.3 g Poly, 0.8 g Sat); 4 mg Cholesterol; 26 g Carbohydrate; 1 g Fibre; 4 g Protein; 132 mg Sodium

CHOICES: 1/2 Fruits; 1/2 Other Choices; 1/2 Milk & Alternatives

---

Paré Pointer

Combine a parrot and a duck, and you'll get a bird that says "Polly want a quacker."

Buttermilk Pancakes and Apples

Tender, sweet apple pieces in a warm maple syrup sauce. Delicious, but serve as an occasional treat.

APPLE TOPPING		
Tart peeled medium apples (such as Granny Smith), cut into 8 wedges each	4	4
Apple juice	1 cup	250 mL
Maple syrup	2 tbsp.	30 mL
Ground cinnamon	1/4 tsp.	1 mL

PANCAKES		
All-purpose flour	1 1/2 cups	375 mL
Baking powder	1 tbsp.	15 mL
Large eggs	2	2
Buttermilk	1 1/4 cups	300 mL
Vanilla	1 tsp.	5 mL

Apple Topping: Combine first 4 ingredients in large frying pan. Heat on medium for about 15 minutes, stirring occasionally, until apples are softened but not broken down, and sauce is slightly thickened. Keep warm. Makes 2 cups (500 mL) topping.

Pancakes: Combine flour and baking powder in large bowl. Make a well in centre.

Beat remaining 3 ingredients in small bowl. Add to well. Stir until just moistened. Heat large non-stick frying pan on medium. Spray lightly with cooking spray. Pour 1/3 cup (75 mL) batter into pan for each pancake. Cook for about 1 minute until bubbles appear on top and edges are dry. Flip. Cook for 1 to 2 minutes until golden. Makes 8 pancakes. Serve topping over pancakes. Serves 4.

1 serving: 341 Calories; 2.9 g Total Fat (trace Mono, 0.1 g Poly, 1.1 g Sat); 113 mg Cholesterol; 70 g Carbohydrate; 2 g Fibre; 10 g Protein; 487 mg Sodium

CHOICES: 2 Grains & Starches; 1 1/2 Fruits; 1/2 Other Choices

Pictured on page 126.

Pear and Yogurt Freeze

A pretty, pale pink "ice" with a hint of pear. Dress up by serving in glass bowls and garnishing with a sprig of mint.

Envelope of unflavoured gelatin (about 1 tbsp., 15 mL)	1/4 oz.	7 g
Cans of pear halves (14 oz., 398 mL, each), drained, juice reserved	2	2
Non-fat berry yogurt	1 1/2 cups	375 mL

Sprinkle gelatin over 1/2 cup (125 mL) pear juice in small saucepan. Let stand for 1 minute. Heat and stir on medium until gelatin is dissolved. Add remaining pear juice. Stir.

Process gelatin mixture, pears and yogurt in blender or food processor until smooth. Spread evenly in ungreased 9 x 13 inch (23 x 33 cm) pan. Freeze, uncovered, for 2 hours. Scrape into large bowl. Beat on high until smooth and slushy. Pour into 1 1/2 quart (1.5 L) airtight container. Freeze until firm. Let stand at room temperature for about 15 minutes before serving. Makes 5 cups (1.25 L).

1/2 cup (125 mL): 62 Calories; 0.1 g Total Fat (trace Mono, trace Poly, 0 g Sat); 0.8 mg Cholesterol; 14 g Carbohydrate; 1 g Fibre; 2 g Protein; 22 mg Sodium

CHOICES: 1/2 Fruits

Pictured on page 126.

Paré Pointer

He is no longer president of the bank—he lost interest.

Peanut Butter Banana Shake

A delicious, creamy shake—perfect for a quick snack or breakfast on the run.

Fat-free sour cream	2/3 cup	150 mL
Medium bananas, sliced	2	2
Light smooth peanut butter	2 tbsp.	30 mL
Ice cubes	3	3

Process first 3 ingredients in blender until smooth.

With motor running, add ice cubes through hole in lid. Process until thick and smooth. Makes 2 cups (500 mL).

1 cup (250 mL): 280 Calories; 6.4 g Total Fat (trace Mono, 0.1 g Poly, 1.4 g Sat); 13 mg Cholesterol; 48 g Carbohydrate; 4 g Fibre; 11 g Protein; 193 mg Sodium

CHOICES: 2 Fruits; 3 Other Choices; 1 Fats

Piñana Milk Smoothie

A smooth, creamy beverage with a refreshing tropical flavour. Great for a quick breakfast or a healthy snack.

Frozen banana, sliced	1	1
Pineapple juice	1 cup	250 mL
Milk	1 cup	250 mL
Vanilla	1/2 tsp.	2 mL

Process all 4 ingredients in blender or food processor until smooth. Serve over ice cubes in tall glasses. Makes 2 1/2 cups (625 mL).

3/4 cup (175 mL): 105 Calories; 0.9 g Total Fat (0.3 g Mono, trace Poly, 0.5 g Sat); 5 mg Cholesterol; 22 g Carbohydrate; 1 g Fibre; 3 g Protein; 41 mg Sodium

CHOICES: 1 Fruits

Pictured on page 144.

HAWAIIAN SMOOTHIE: Omit vanilla. Add 1 tsp. (5 mL) coconut extract.

Strawberry Orange Smoothie

A creamy drink with refreshing strawberry and orange flavours. A great mid-morning or mid-afternoon pick-me-up.

Milk	1 cup	250 mL
Vanilla frozen yogurt	1/2 cup	125 mL
Frozen concentrated orange juice	1/4 cup	60 mL
Large fresh strawberries	8	8

Process all 4 ingredients in blender or food processor for about 30 seconds until smooth. Makes 3 cups (750 mL).

3/4 cup (175 mL): 105 Calories; 1.9 g Total Fat (0.3 g Mono, 0.1 g Poly, 1.1 g Sat); 8 mg Cholesterol; 19 g Carbohydrate; 1 g Fibre; 4 g Protein; 45 mg Sodium

CHOICES: 1/2 Fruits; 1/2 Milk & Alternatives

Pictured on page 144.

Variation: Use frozen strawberries instead of fresh. With blender motor running, drop frozen strawberries, 1 at a time, through hole in lid and blend until mixture is thick and smooth.

1. Roasted Cauliflower, page 103
2. Pea Medley, page 110
3. Maple Butternut Squash, page 104
4. Oven-Fried Vegetables, page 111

Props courtesy of: Pier 1 Imports

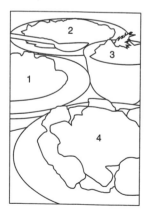

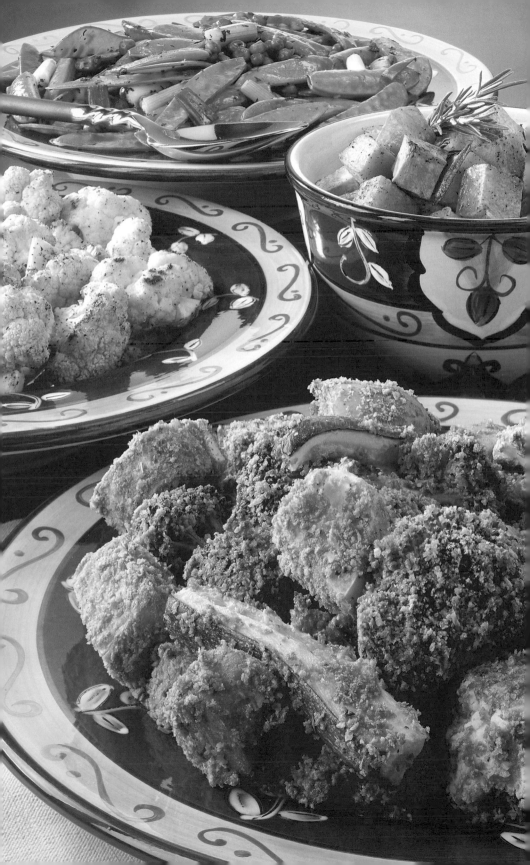

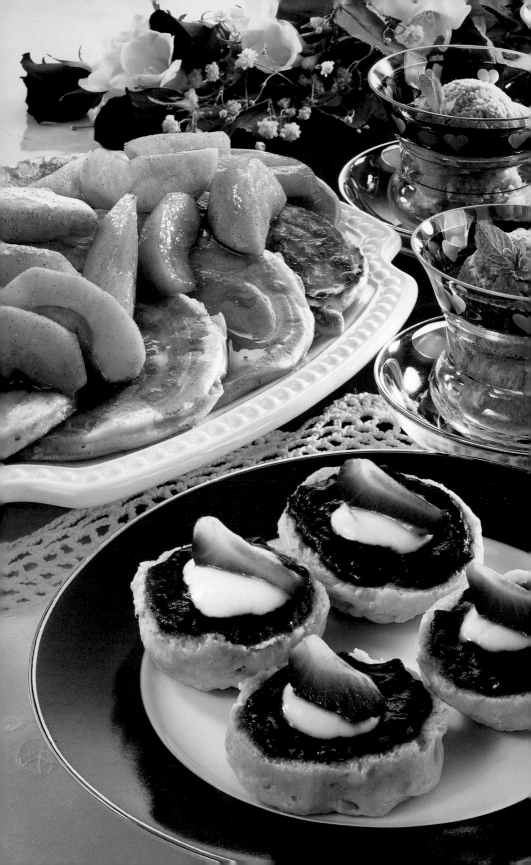

Corn Muffin Surprise

A ribbon of strawberry jam runs through these tasty muffins.

Yellow cornmeal	1 cup	250 mL
Buttermilk	1 cup	250 mL
Whole-wheat flour	1/2 cup	125 mL
All-purpose flour	1/2 cup	125 mL
Brown sugar, packed	2 tbsp.	30 mL
Baking powder	1 tbsp.	15 mL
Salt	1/4 tsp.	1 mL
Large egg	1	1
Canola oil	2 tbsp.	30 mL
Unsweetened strawberry jam	8 tsp.	40 mL

Combine cornmeal and buttermilk in small bowl. Let stand for 15 minutes.

Combine next 5 ingredients in medium bowl. Make a well in centre.

Beat egg and canola oil with fork in small cup until frothy. Add to well. Add cornmeal mixture. Stir until just combined. Grease 8 muffin cups with cooking spray. Spoon about 1/4 cup (60 mL) batter into each cup.

Drop 1 tsp. (5 mL) jam into centre of each muffin. Spoon remaining batter over jam. Pour about 1/4 inch (6 mm) water into empty muffin cups before baking muffins. Bake in 400°F (205°C) oven for about 15 minutes until golden and top springs back when pressed. Let stand in pan for 5 minutes before removing to wire rack to cool. Makes 8 muffins.

1 muffin: 184 Calories; 4.8 g Total Fat (2.1 g Mono, 1.2 g Poly, 0.7 g Sat); 29 mg Cholesterol; 32 g Carbohydrate; 2 g Fibre; 5 g Protein; 535 mg Sodium

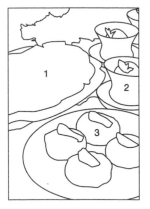

CHOICES: 1 1/2 Grains & Starches; 1/2 Fats

1. Buttermilk Pancakes and Apples, page 121
2. Pear and Yogurt Freeze, page 122
3. Strawberry Shortcakes, page 119

Props courtesy of: Pier 1 Imports

Breakfast Muffins

A simple breakfast muffin with the sweet taste of dates and apples. Great for a meal on the go or a lunch box snack.

All-purpose flour	1 1/4 cups	300 mL
Brown sugar, packed	2/3 cup	150 mL
Whole-wheat flour	1/2 cup	125 mL
Bran flakes cereal	1/3 cup	75 mL
Baking powder	1 tbsp.	15 mL
Chopped pitted dates	1 cup	250 mL
Chopped dried apple	1/2 cup	125 mL
Large egg	1	1
Buttermilk	3/4 cup	175 mL
Unsweetened applesauce	1/3 cup	75 mL
Finely grated orange zest	1 tsp.	5 mL

Combine first 5 ingredients in large bowl.

Add dates and apple. Mix well. Make a well in centre.

Beat egg with fork in small bowl. Add remaining 3 ingredients. Stir. Add to well. Stir until just moistened. Grease 12 muffin cups with cooking spray. Fill cups 3/4 full. Bake in 375°F (190°C) oven for about 20 minutes until wooden pick inserted in centre of muffin comes out clean. Let stand in pan for 5 minutes before removing to wire rack to cool. Makes 12 muffins.

1 muffin: 185 Calories; 0.7 g Total Fat (trace Mono, trace Poly, 0.2 g Sat); 18.9 mg Cholesterol; 43 g Carbohydrate; 3 g Fibre; 4 g Protein; 218 mg Sodium

CHOICES: 1 Grains & Starches; 1 Fruits; 1 Other Choices

Apple Gingerbread Mini-Muffins

A moist muffin with well-balanced flavours. Distinct spices add to the sweet apple and molasses flavours. Great for a pop-in-your-mouth snack.

Diced peeled apple	1 cup	250 mL
Lemon juice	1 tsp.	5 mL
All-purpose flour	3/4 cup	175 mL
Whole wheat flour	3/4 cup	175 mL
Brown sugar, packed	1/4 cup	60 mL
Ground ginger	1 1/2 tsp.	7 mL
Ground allspice	1/4 tsp.	1 mL
Large egg	1	1
Egg white (large)	1	1
Fancy (mild) molasses	1/3 cup	75 mL
Buttermilk	1/4 cup	60 mL
Canola oil	3 tbsp.	50 mL
Baking soda	3/4 tsp.	4 mL

Combine apple and lemon juice in small bowl.

Combine next 5 ingredients in medium bowl. Make a well in centre. Add apple mixture to well. Do not stir.

Beat remaining 6 ingredients in same small bowl until combined. Add to apple mixture. Stir until just moistened. Spoon 1 rounded teaspoonful into each of 24 well-greased mini-muffin cups. Bake in 375°F (190°C) oven for about 10 minutes until wooden pick inserted in centre of muffin comes out clean. Let stand in pan for 2 minutes before removing to wire rack to cool. Makes 24 mini-muffins.

1 muffin: 69 Calories; 2.1 g Total Fat (1.0 g Mono, 0.5 g Poly, 0.2 g Sat); 9 mg Cholesterol; 12 g Carbohydrate; 1 g Fibre; 1 g Protein; 50 mg Sodium

CHOICES: 1/2 Other Choices

Pictured on page 144.

APPLE GINGERBREAD MUFFINS: Spoon batter into 12 well-greased regular-sized muffin cups. Bake in 375°F (190°C) oven for about 20 minutes until wooden pick inserted in centre of muffin comes out clean. Let stand in pan for 5 minutes before removing to wire rack to cool. Makes 12 muffins.

1 muffin: 139 Calories; 4.1 g Total Fat (2.0 g Mono, 1.1 g Poly, 0.4 g Sat); 18 mg Cholesterol; 24 g Carbohydrate; 1 g Fibre; 3 g Protein; 100 mg Sodium

CHOICES: 1/2 Grains & Starches; 1/2 Other Choices; 1/2 Fats

Cheesy Pocket Puffs

These attractive, golden crescents have a warm, cheese filling. Great with Corn Yogurt Dip, page 142.

Whole-wheat flour	1 cup	250 mL
All-purpose flour	1 cup	250 mL
Instant yeast	2 tsp.	10 mL
Salt	1/4 tsp.	1 mL
Very warm water	3/4 cup	175 mL
Olive oil	1 tbsp.	15 mL
Granulated sugar	1 tsp.	5 mL
CHEESY FILLING		
Mashed non-fat cottage cheese	2/3 cup	150 mL
Crumbled low-fat feta cheese (about 3 oz., 85 g)	2/3 cup	150 mL
Finely chopped green onion	1 tbsp.	15 mL
Finely chopped fresh dill (or 1/4 tsp., 1 mL, dill weed)	1 tsp.	5 mL
Garlic powder	1/8 tsp.	0.5 mL
Pepper, sprinkle		
Sesame seeds	1 tsp.	15 mL

Put first 4 ingredients into food processor fitted with dough blade.

Stir next 3 ingredients in liquid measure until sugar is dissolved. With motor running, pour mixture through feed chute. Process for 30 to 40 seconds until dough comes together and ball begins to form. Place dough in greased bowl, turning once to grease top. Cover with greased waxed paper and tea towel. Let stand in oven with light on and door closed for about 30 minutes until starting to rise.

Cheesy Filling: Mix first 6 ingredients in small bowl until creamy. Makes 1 cup (250 mL) filling.

Punch dough down. Divide into 8 portions. Lightly grease work surface with cooking spray. Roll out 1 portion of dough to 3 1/2 inch (9 cm) circle. Cover remaining portions to keep from drying out. Place about 2 tbsp. (30 mL) filling on half of circle. Dampen edge of circle with water. Fold dough over. Pinch edges together to seal. Place on lightly greased baking sheet. Repeat with remaining portions of dough and filling.

(continued on next page)

Lightly spray surface of puffs with cooking spray. Sprinkle with sesame seeds. Cover with tea towel. Let stand in oven with light on and door closed for about 1 hour until doubled in size. Bake in 375°F (190°C) oven for about 15 minutes until golden. Remove to wire rack to cool. Makes 8 puffs.

1 puff: 154 Calories; 3.4 g Total Fat (1.3 g Mono, 0.4 g Poly, 1.1 g Sat); 5 mg Cholesterol; 24 g Carbohydrate; 2 g Fibre; 8 g Protein; 281 mg Sodium

CHOICES: 1 1/2 Grains & Starches; 1/2 Meat & Alternatives

Pumpkin and Fig Muffins

A moist, soft-crumb muffin with a delicate pumpkin flavour. The figs add a wonderful sweetness and texture.

All-purpose flour	1 cup	250 mL
Whole-wheat flour	3/4 cup	175 mL
Dark brown sugar, packed	1/2 cup	125 mL
Baking powder	2 tbsp.	30 mL
Ground cinnamon	3/4 tsp.	4 mL
Ground nutmeg	1/2 tsp.	2 mL
Ground ginger	1/2 tsp.	2 mL
Milk	1 cup	250 mL
Canned pure pumpkin (no spices)	2/3 cup	150 mL
Canola oil	3 tbsp.	50 mL
Egg whites (large)	2	2
Chopped dried figs	1/2 cup	125 mL

Combine first 7 ingredients in large bowl. Make a well in centre.

Beat next 4 ingredients in medium bowl until smooth. Pour into well.

Add figs. Stir until just moistened. Grease 12 muffin cups with cooking spray. Fill cups 3/4 full. Bake in 400°F (205°C) oven for about 18 minutes until wooden pick inserted in centre of muffin comes out clean. Let stand in pan for 5 minutes before removing to wire rack to cool. Makes 12 muffins.

1 muffin: 154 Calories; 4.0 g Total Fat (2.1 g Mono, 1.1 g Poly, 0.5 g Sat); 1 mg Cholesterol; 27 g Carbohydrate; 2 g Fibre; 4 g Protein; 300 mg Sodium

CHOICES: 1 Grains & Starches; 1/2 Other Choices; 1/2 Fats

Carrot Cheese Muffins

A sweet coconut and cream cheese filling bursts through the tops of these spiced carrot muffins. Kids will love them for a snack or for breakfast.

All-purpose flour	3/4 cup	175 mL
Whole-wheat flour	3/4 cup	175 mL
Brown sugar, packed	1/2 cup	125 mL
Baking powder	1 tsp.	5 mL
Baking soda	1 tsp.	5 mL
Ground cinnamon	1 tsp.	5 mL
Ground ginger	1/2 tsp.	2 mL
Salt	1/4 tsp.	1 mL
Ground nutmeg	1/8 tsp.	0.5 mL
Large egg	1	1
Light sour cream	3/4 cup	175 mL
Canola oil	3 tbsp.	50 mL
Finely shredded carrot	1 cup	250 mL
Chopped raisins	1/2 cup	125 mL
Vanilla	1 tsp.	5 mL
COCONUT CHEESE FILLING		
Light spreadable cream cheese	1/3 cup	75 mL
Flaked coconut, toasted (see Tip, page 97)	1/4 cup	60 mL
Icing (confectioner's) sugar	2 tbsp.	30 mL
Vanilla	1/4 tsp.	1 mL

Combine first 9 ingredients in large bowl. Make a well in centre.

Beat next 3 ingredients in medium bowl. Add next 3 ingredients. Stir. Add to well. Stir until just moistened. Grease 12 muffin cups with cooking spray. Fill cups 3/4 full.

Coconut Cheese Filling: Combine all 4 ingredients in small bowl. Gently press 2 tsp. (10 mL) mixture down into centre of each muffin. Bake in 400°F (205°C) oven for about 15 minutes until golden. Let stand in pan for 5 minutes before removing to wire rack to cool. Makes 12 muffins.

1 muffin: 189 Calories; 6.3 g Total Fat (2.0 g Mono, 1.1 g Poly, 1.9 g Sat); 25 mg Cholesterol; 30 g Carbohydrate; 2 g Fibre; 4 g Protein; 272 mg Sodium

CHOICES: 1/2 Grains & Starches; 1/2 Fruits; 1 Other Choices; 1 Fats

Pictured on page 144.

Date and Orange Loaf

This perfectly risen loaf has a great appearance and texture once sliced. The orange zest creates a wonderfully complementary flavour to the dates. Delicious!

All-purpose flour	2 1/2 cups	625 mL
Granulated sugar	3/4 cup	175 mL
Baking powder	1 1/2 tbsp.	25 mL
Hard margarine (or butter)	1/3 cup	75 mL
Mllk	1 cup	250 mL
Large eggs, fork-beaten	2	2
Finely grated orange zest	1 1/2 tsp.	7 mL
Chopped pitted dates	1 cup	250 mL

Combine first 3 ingredients in large bowl. Make a well in centre.

Melt margarine in small saucepan on medium. Remove from heat. Add milk. Stir. Add eggs and zest. Stir. Add to well.

Add dates. Stir until combined. Spread evenly in greased 9 x 5 x 3 inch (23 x 12.5 x 7.5 cm) loaf pan. Bake in 350°F (175°C) oven for 55 to 60 minutes until wooden pick inserted in centre comes out clean. Let stand in pan for 10 minutes before removing to wire rack to cool. Cuts into 16 slices.

1 slice: 181 Calories; 4.4 g Total Fat (0.1 g Mono, 0.0 g Poly, 1.0 g Sat); 28 mg Cholesterol; 33 g Carbohydrate; 1 g Fibre; 3 g Protein; 206 mg Sodium

CHOICES: 1 Grains & Starches; 1/2 Fruits; 1/2 Other Choices; 1/2 Fats

Pictured on page 144.

Pumpkin Bread

Moist, pumpkin-flavoured squares with a subtle hint of orange.

Granulated sugar	1/3 cup	75 mL
Hard margarine (or butter), softened	1/4 cup	60 mL
Can of pure pumpkin (no spices)	14 oz.	398 mL
Large eggs	2	2
Egg white (large)	1	1
Finely grated orange zest	2 tsp.	10 mL
All-purpose flour	1 1/4 cups	300 mL
Chopped pecans, toasted (see Tip, page 97)	1/3 cup	75 mL
Baking powder	4 tsp.	20 mL
Ground cinnamon	1/2 tsp.	2 mL
Ground nutmeg	1/4 tsp.	1 mL
Salt	1/4 tsp.	1 mL

Beat sugar and margarine in large bowl until light and creamy.

Add next 4 ingredients. Beat until well combined.

Combine remaining 6 ingredients in medium bowl. Add to pumpkin mixture. Stir. Spread evenly in greased 8 x 8 inch (20 x 20 cm) pan. Bake in 350°F (175°C) oven for about 45 minutes until wooden pick inserted in centre comes out clean. Let stand in pan for 10 minutes before removing to wire rack to cool. Cuts into 16 pieces.

1 piece: 111 Calories; 5.2 g Total Fat (1.0 g Mono, 0.5 g Poly, 0.9 g Sat); 27 mg Cholesterol; 14 g Carbohydrate; 1 g Fibre; 2 g Protein; 213 mg Sodium

CHOICES: 1 Grains & Starches; 1 Fats

Kid-Friendly Idea: Omit pecans.

1 piece: 94 Calories; 3.4 g Total Fat (trace Mono, 0 g Poly, 1 g Sat); 27 mg Cholesterol; 14 g Carbohydrate; 1 g Fibre; 2 g Protein; 213 mg Sodium

CHOICES: 1/2 Grains & Starches; 1/2 Fats

Peanut Butter Cookies

Golden morsels with a classic peanut butter cookie appearance. This immensely satisfying snack has a mild peanut butter flavour.

Light smooth peanut butter	1/2 cup	125 mL
Brown sugar, packed	1/3 cup	75 mL
Hard margarine (or butter), softened	1/4 cup	60 mL
Large egg	1	1
Milk	1/4 cup	60 mL
Vanilla	1/2 tsp.	2 mL
All-purpose flour	1 1/2 cups	375 mL
Baking powder	1/2 tsp.	2 mL
Baking soda	1/2 tsp.	2 mL

Beat first 3 ingredients in small bowl until light and creamy.

Add next 3 ingredients. Beat until well combined.

Combine remaining 3 ingredients in medium bowl. Add to margarine mixture. Mix well. Drop by slightly rounded tablespoonfuls, about 2 inches (5 cm) apart, onto greased baking sheet. Press with fork to flatten slightly. Bake in 375°F (190°C) oven for about 12 minutes until lightly golden. Let stand on baking sheet for 10 minutes before removing to wire rack to cool. Makes about 30 cookies.

1 cookie: 72 Calories; 3.2 g Total Fat (trace Mono, 0 g Poly, 0.7 g Sat); 7 mg Cholesterol; 9 g Carbohydrate; trace Fibre; 2 g Protein; 82 mg Sodium

CHOICES: 1/2 Fats

Pictured on page 144.

Tropical Ice Pops

The complementary flavours of banana and citrus fruits combine in these oh-so-refreshing pops. A delicious treat to enjoy on a summer day.

Can of crushed pineapple	14 oz.	398 mL
Mashed banana (about 2 medium)	1 cup	250 mL
Orange juice	1 cup	250 mL
Lime juice	1 tbsp.	15 mL
Plastic cups (5 oz., 142 mL, size), see Note	14	14
Freezer pop sticks	14	14

Combine first 4 ingredients in large bowl. Pour into 9 x 9 inch (23 x 23 cm) pan lined with plastic wrap. Freeze for about 1 hour until almost set. Process mixture in blender or food processor until smooth and creamy.

Spoon mixture into cups. Insert freezer pop stick into centre of each. Freeze for about 6 hours until firm. Dip cups into warm water briefly before turning out. Makes 14 ice pops.

1 ice pop: 47 Calories; 0.1 g Total Fat (trace Mono, trace Poly, trace Sat); 0 mg Cholesterol; 12 g Carbohydrate; 1 g Fibre; trace Protein; 1 mg Sodium

Note: Ice pops can also be made in 14 ice pop molds or small waxed cups if you have them.

CHOICES: 1 Fruits

Chewy Banana Nuggets

Soft, moist bites with a natural banana sweetness and a toasted coconut flavour. A healthy combination of ingredients that is great as a snack or as a light dessert.

Medium bananas	3	3
Lemon juice	1 tbsp.	15 mL
Medium unsweetened coconut	1 1/2 cups	375 mL
Finely chopped pitted dates	1 cup	250 mL
Quick-cooking rolled oats	1/2 cup	125 mL
Vanilla	1 tsp.	5 mL
Ground cinnamon	1/2 tsp.	2 mL

Mash bananas and lemon juice in large bowl until smooth.

Add remaining 5 ingredients. Stir until moistened. Drop by 2 tsp. (10 mL) spoonfuls onto greased baking sheet. Bake on rack just above centre in 325°F (160°C) oven for about 30 minutes until dry and golden. Makes about 60 nuggets.

1 nugget: 29 Calories; 1.3 g Total Fat (0.1 g Mono, trace Poly, 1.1 g Sat); 0 mg Cholesterol; 4 g Carbohydrate; 1 g Fibre; 0.4 g Protein; 1 mg Sodium

CHOICES: No Choices

Paré Pointer

Eating soup is a real strain when you have a big bushy moustache.

Fruity Granola Bars

Toasted oatmeal and coconut give a nutty flavour to these soft, fruity snack bars. Great for snacks or as a nutritious breakfast food. Kids will love them.

Quick-cooking rolled oats	5 cups	1.25 L
Flaked coconut	3/4 cup	175 mL
Can of low-fat sweetened condensed milk	11 oz.	300 mL
Unsweetened applesauce	2/3 cup	150 mL
Tub margarine, melted	1/4 cup	60 mL
Canola oil	1/4 cup	60 mL
Liquid honey	1/4 cup	60 mL
Dried cranberries	1 cup	250 mL
Finely chopped dried apricots	1 cup	250 mL

Combine rolled oats and coconut in medium bowl. Spread on ungreased baking sheet. Bake in 350°F (175°C) oven for 15 to 20 minutes, stirring every 5 minutes, until fragrant and coconut is golden.

Mix next 5 ingredients in large bowl until well combined. Add rolled oats mixture. Stir until moistened.

Add cranberries and apricots. Stir until well distributed. Line 9 x 13 inch (23 x 33 cm) pan with foil, leaving 1 inch (2.5 cm) overhang on long sides. Spray well with cooking spray. Transfer oat mixture to pan. Pack down firmly. Bake in 325°F (160°C) oven for about 45 minutes until set and golden. Cool completely. Using foil overhang, lift mixture from pan. Carefully peel off and discard foil. Cut mixture lengthwise into thirds. Cut each third into ten 1 1/4 inch (3 cm) wide bars. Wipe blade of knife or run under hot water between each cut. Wrap bars individually in plastic wrap. Store at room temperature or place bars in resealable freezer bag to freeze for longer storage. Makes 30 bars.

1 bar: 163 Calories; 5.3 g Total Fat (1.1 g Mono, 0.5 g Poly, 1.2 g Sat); 1 mg Cholesterol; 26 g Carbohydrate; 2 g Fibre; 3 g Protein; 33 mg Sodium

CHOICES: 1 Grains & Starches; 1/2 Fruits; 1/2 Milk & Alternatives; 1 Fats

Pictured on page 144.

Chilled Oatmeal Bars

Delicious, nutty granola bars with a variety of healthy ingredients. A substantial snack that is perfect for eating on the go.

Light smooth peanut butter	1/2 cup	125 mL
Hard margarine (or butter), softened	2 tbsp.	30 mL
Liquid honey	2 tbsp.	30 mL
Large eggs, fork-beaten	2	2
Vanilla	1 tsp.	5 mL
Quick-cooking rolled oats	2 cups	500 mL
Sliced natural almonds	1/2 cup	125 mL
Unsalted sunflower seeds	1/4 cup	60 mL
Raw pumpkin seeds	1/4 cup	60 mL

Combine first 3 ingredients in large saucepan. Heat and stir on medium until smooth. Remove from heat.

Add eggs and vanilla. Beat with fork or whisk until slightly thickened.

Add remaining 4 ingredients. Stir until coated. Line 9 x 9 inch (23 x 23 cm) pan with foil, leaving 1 inch (2.5 cm) overhang on 2 sides. Transfer oat mixture to pan. Pack down firmly. Chill for about 4 hours until firm. Using foil overhang, lift mixture from pan. Carefully peel off foil and discard. Cuts into 36 bars.

1 bar: 75 Calories; 4.4 g Total Fat (0.8 g Mono, 0.8 g Poly, 0.7 g Sat); 12 mg Cholesterol; 7 g Carbohydrate; 1 g Fibre; 3 g Protein; 38 mg Sodium

CHOICES: 1/2 Fats

Variation: After packing down oat mixture in pan lined with greased foil, bake in 350°F (175°) oven for about 20 minutes until golden. Let stand on wire rack until cool.

 To store granola bar-type bars, cut and wrap in plastic wrap. Keep a supply in either the refrigerator or the freezer for a ready-made "snack bar." Great for bag lunches or after-school snacks.

Pizza Swirls

*These whole-wheat pinwheels make a great snack. Wrap the swirls
individually in plastic wrap for a take-along treat. Good warm or cold.*

All-purpose flour	1 cup	250 mL
Whole-wheat flour	1 cup	250 mL
Baking powder	1 tbsp.	15 mL
Dried basil	1/2 tsp.	2 mL
Dried oregano	1/4 tsp.	1 mL
Salt	1/4 tsp.	1 mL
Skim milk	1/2 cup	125 mL
Olive oil	1/3 cup	75 mL
Yellow cornmeal	1 tbsp.	15 mL
Pizza sauce	1/2 cup	125 mL
Diced red (or yellow) pepper	1/2 cup	125 mL
Diced no-fat deli ham slices	1 cup	250 mL
Grated part-skim mozzarella cheese	1 cup	250 mL
Finely grated fresh Parmesan cheese	2 tbsp.	30 mL

Combine first 6 ingredients in large bowl. Make a well in centre.

Pour milk and olive oil into well. Stir until ball starts to form. Turn out onto
lightly floured surface. Knead 8 times.

Sprinkle cornmeal over 10 x 20 inch (25 x 50 cm) work surface. Roll out
dough over cornmeal to 8 x 18 inch (20 x 46 cm) rectangle.

Spread pizza sauce over dough, leaving 1/4 inch (6 mm) border around edge.

Combine remaining 4 ingredients in medium bowl. Scatter evenly
over pizza sauce. Roll up, jelly roll-style, from long side. Dough will be
somewhat stiff. Pinch edge against roll to seal, leaving ends open. Slice into
twenty 1 inch (2.5 cm) thick rounds. Arrange, cut-side down, about 1 inch
(2.5 cm) apart on greased baking sheet. Bake in 425°F (220°C) oven for
about 10 minutes until starting to turn golden. Let stand on baking sheet
for 5 minutes before removing to wire rack to cool. Makes 20 swirls.

*1 swirl: 114 Calories; 5.6 g Total Fat (2.7 g Mono, 0.6 g Poly, 1.5 g Sat); 7 mg Cholesterol;
11 g Carbohydrate; 1 g Fibre; 5 g Protein; 457 mg Sodium*

CHOICES: 1/2 Grains & Starches; 1/2 Fats

Parmesan Chicken Fingers

These flavourful fingers are ready in about 30 minutes. May be frozen after cooking and reheated in the microwave or oven. They're even good cold—one batch will go a long way for snacking!

Boneless, skinless chicken breast halves	1 lb.	454 g
Non-fat plain yogurt	1/2 cup	125 mL
Garlic and herb no-salt seasoning	1 tsp.	5 mL
Paprika	1/2 tsp.	2 mL
Garlic powder	1/4 tsp.	1 mL
Lemon pepper	1/4 tsp.	1 mL
Finely grated fresh Parmesan cheese	2/3 cup	150 mL
Fine dry bread crumbs	2/3 cup	150 mL
Chopped fresh parsley	2 tsp.	10 mL
(or 1/2 tsp., 2 mL, flakes)		

Cut each chicken breast lengthwise into 6 or 7 strips.

Combine next 5 ingredients in medium bowl. Add chicken. Stir until coated. Cover. Marinate in refrigerator for at least 1 hour.

Combine remaining 3 ingredients in shallow dish. Remove chicken strips from marinade, 1 at a time, making sure to leave some yogurt mixture on each. Press both sides of strips into cheese mixture until coated. Arrange in single layer on well-greased baking sheet. Spray chicken with cooking spray. Bake in 425°F (220°C) oven for 15 to 20 minutes until no longer pink inside. Serve hot or cold. Serves 8.

1 serving: 128 Calories; 3.1 g Total Fat (0.2 g Mono, 0.2 g Poly, 1.2 g Sat); 38 mg Cholesterol; 6 g Carbohydrate; trace Fibre; 18 g Protein; 229 mg Sodium

CHOICES: 1 Meat & Alternatives

Pictured on page 143.

Corn Yogurt Dip

The creamy cheese and sweet corn flavours in this dip will appeal to children and adults alike. Serve warm with fresh, crisp veggies, such as carrot sticks, cucumber pieces, celery sticks, radishes or cauliflower florets.

Corn relish	1/2 cup	125 mL
Low-fat plain yogurt	1/2 cup	125 mL
Grated light sharp Cheddar cheese	1/3 cup	75 mL
Chopped fresh chives	2 tbsp.	30 mL

Combine all 4 ingredients in small saucepan. Heat and stir on medium for 5 to 6 minutes until cheese is melted. Makes 1 cup (250 mL).

2 tbsp. (30 mL): 34 Calories; 1.0 g Total Fat (trace Mono, trace Poly, 0.6 g Sat); 3 mg Cholesterol; 5 g Carbohydrate; trace Fibre; 2 g Protein; 41 mg Sodium

CHOICES: No Choices

Pictured at right.

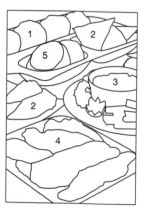

1. Pepper Cheese Muffins, page 150
2. Chicken Samosas, page 146
3. Corn Yogurt Dip, above
4. Parmesan Chicken Fingers, page 141
5. Pesto Cheese Spirals, page 149

Props courtesy of: Stokes
The Bay

Snacks

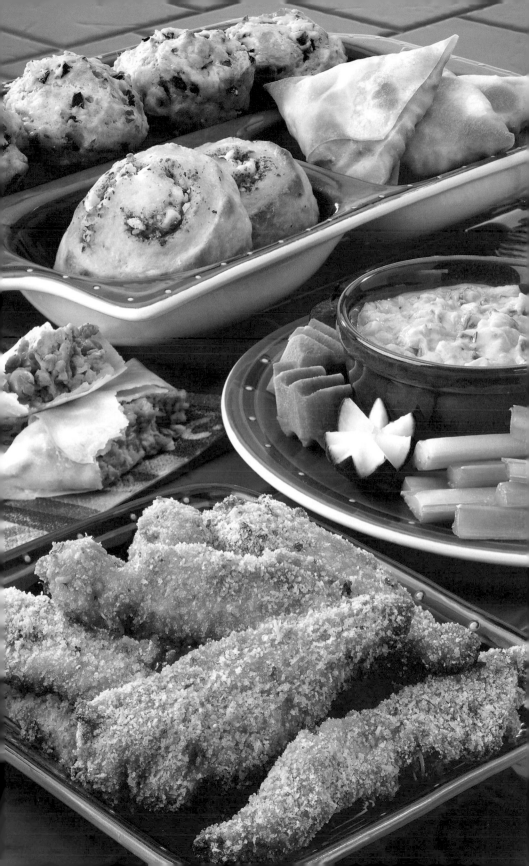

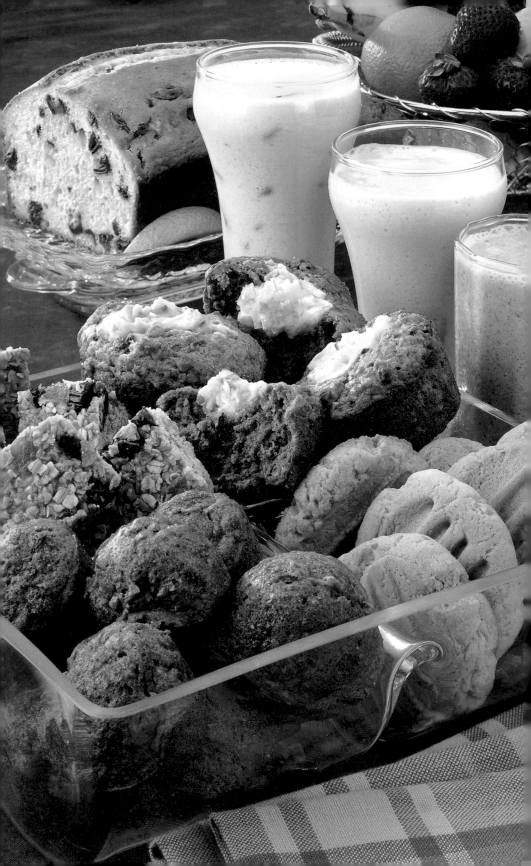

Ham and Melon Skewers

Perfectly woven flavours on a refreshing summer kabob.

Small cantaloupe	1	1
Fat-free deli ham slices	4	4
Bamboo skewers (4 inch, 10 cm, length), or cocktail picks	12	12

Cut cantaloupe in half. Scoop out and discard seeds and pulp. Cut each half into 6 wedges. Cut off and discard rind. Cut each wedge crosswise into 3 pieces, for a total of 36 pieces.

Cut each ham slice lengthwise into 3 strips.

Thread 3 cantaloupe pieces alternately with 1 ham strip onto each skewer. Repeat with remaining cantaloupe, ham and skewers. Makes 12 skewers.

1 skewer: 20 Calories; 0.3 g Total Fat (0.1 g Mono, 0.1 g Poly, 0.1 g Sat); 3 mg Cholesterol; 3 g Carbohydrate; trace Fibre; 1 g Protein; 93 mg Sodium

CHOICES: No Choices

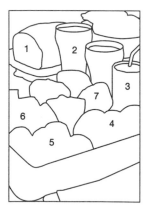

1. Date and Orange Loaf, page 133
2. Piñana Milk Smoothie, page 123
3. Strawberry Orange Smoothie, page 124
4. Peanut Butter Cookies, page 135
5. Apple Gingerbread Mini-Muffins, page 129
6. Fruity Granola Bars, page 138
7. Carrot Cheese Muffins, page 132

Props courtesy of: Pier 1 Imports
Danesco Inc.
Canhome Global

Chicken Samosas

Pronounced sah-MOH-sahs, these crisp pastries are filled with tender chicken and cooked vegetables. Good as is or dipped in sweet chili sauce, chutney, plum sauce or ketchup.

CHICKEN FILLING

Olive oil	1 tbsp.	15 mL
Finely chopped onion	2 cups	500 mL
Lean ground chicken	1 lb.	454 g
Lemon pepper (optional)	1/2 tsp.	2 mL
Garlic cloves, minced	2	2
(or 1/2 tsp., 2 mL, powder)		
Diced peeled potato	1/4 lb.	113 g
Frozen peas	2/3 cup	150 mL
Low-sodium prepared chicken broth	1/2 cup	125 mL
Grated carrot	1/3 cup	75 mL
Garlic and herb no-salt seasoning	1 1/2 tsp.	7 mL
(such as Mrs. Dash)		
All-purpose flour	2 tbsp.	30 mL
Water	3 tbsp.	50 mL
Samosa wrappers (see Note)	18	18

Chicken Filling: Heat olive oil in large saucepan on medium. Add onion. Cook for 5 to 10 minutes, stirring often, until onion is soft and golden.

Add next 3 ingredients. Cook on medium for about 5 minutes, stirring constantly, until chicken is broken up and no pink remains.

Add next 5 ingredients. Stir. Bring to a boil. Reduce heat to medium. Cover. Cook for 15 to 20 minutes, stirring occasionally, until potato is tender. Remove cover. Increase heat if necessary to boil off any remaining moisture. Cool.

Stir flour into water in small cup until consistency of smooth paste.

(continued on next page)

Lay 1 samosa wrapper on work surface (diagram 1). Fold according to diagrams 2 to 5, moistening edges of wrapper with flour mixture. Turn over. Spoon 3 tbsp. (50 mL) chicken filling into pocket. Moisten flaps with flour mixture (diagram 6). Fold to seal (diagram 7). Arrange, seam-side down, on greased baking sheet. Repeat with remaining wrappers, flour mixture and filling. Spray samosas lightly with cooking spray. Bake in 400°F (205°C) oven for about 15 minutes until crisp and lightly golden. Makes 18 samosas.

1 samosa: 193 Calories; 6.8 g Total Fat (0.6 g Mono, 0.1 g Poly, 1.7 g Sat); 17 mg Cholesterol; 26 g Carbohydrate; 1 g Fibre; 8 g Protein; 367 mg Sodium

CHOICES: 1 1/2 Grains & Starches

Pictured on page 143.

Note: Samosa wrappers can be found in the freezer sections of large grocery stores or East Indian markets.

To Make Ahead: Prepare to baking stage. Wrap individually in plastic wrap and freeze. Bake in 400°F (205°C) oven for about 15 minutes until crisp and lightly golden. Or bake before freezing and reheat in microwave.

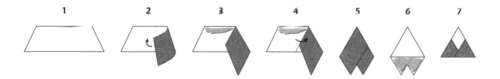

Cheese Tortillas

Crisp tortillas with a spicy cheese topping. Best served warm.

Light spreadable cream cheese	1/2 cup	125 mL
Chili sauce	1 tbsp.	15 mL
Low-sodium soy sauce	1 tbsp.	15 mL
Whole-wheat flour tortillas (10 inch, 25 cm, diameter)	2	2
Sesame seeds	2 tsp.	10 mL

Combine first 3 ingredients in small bowl.

Place tortillas on ungreased baking sheet. Spread cream cheese mixture over tortillas.

Sprinkle with sesame seeds. Bake in 425°F (220°C) oven for about 10 minutes until tortillas are crisp. Cut each into 8 wedges. Makes 16 wedges.

2 wedges: 62 Calories; 3.0 g Total Fat (trace Mono, 0.1 g Poly, 1.8 g Sat); 8 mg Cholesterol; 7 g Carbohydrate; 1 g Fibre; 3 g Protein; 248 mg Sodium

CHOICES: 1/2 Grains & Starches; 1/2 Fats

Paré Pointer
Crooked dough makes money—that's why pretzel sellers do so well.

Pesto Cheese Spirals

Scrumptious! These easy, fluffy biscuits are spiralled with basil pesto. Freeze in a sealed container and enjoy them thawed to room temperature, or reheat from frozen by covering with foil and baking in 450°F (230°C) oven for 15 to 20 minutes until warmed.

All-purpose flour	2 1/4 cups	550 mL
Baking powder	1 tbsp.	15 mL
Granulated sugar	1 tbsp.	15 mL
Hard margarine (or butter)	1 tbsp.	15 mL
Buttermilk, approximately	1 cup	250 mL
Basil pesto	1/3 cup	75 mL
Crumbled low-fat feta cheese	1/2 cup	125 mL

Combine first 3 ingredients in large bowl. Cut in margarine until consistency of coarse crumbs.

Stir in enough buttermilk to make soft, sticky dough. Turn out onto lightly floured surface. Knead about 8 times until smooth. Roll out dough to 6 x 12 inch (15 x 30 cm) rectangle.

Spread pesto over dough. Sprinkle with cheese. Roll up, jelly roll-style, from long side. Pinch edge against roll to seal. Cut into 12 slices, about 1 inch (2.5 cm) thick. Arrange, cut-side down, about 2 inches (5 cm) apart, on greased baking sheet. Bake in 475°F (240°C) oven for about 15 minutes until edges are lightly browned. Let stand on baking sheet for 5 minutes before removing to wire rack to cool. Makes 12 spirals.

1 spiral: 145 Calories; 5.2 g Total Fat (0 g Mono, 0 g Poly, 1.3 g Sat); 5 mg Cholesterol; 20 g Carbohydrate; trace Fibre; 5 g Protein; 305 mg Sodium

CHOICES: 1 Grains & Starches; 1 Fats

Pictured on page 143.

Pepper Cheese Muffins

*A savoury muffin speckled with red peppers, green basil and orange cheese.
Red peppers may be roasted under the broiler, on the barbecue, or purchased
in a jar and drained.*

Canola oil	1 tsp.	5 mL
Chopped onion	1 cup	250 mL
Garlic clove, minced	1	1
(or 1/4 tsp., 1 mL, powder)		
All-purpose flour	2 1/2 cups	625 mL
Baking powder	1 tbsp.	15 mL
Chopped roasted red pepper, blotted dry	1 cup	250 mL
Grated light sharp Cheddar cheese	1/2 cup	125 mL
Chopped fresh basil	2 tbsp.	30 mL
(or 1 1/2 tsp., 7 mL, dried)		
Chili paste (sambal oelek)	1/2 tsp.	2 mL
Pepper	1/4 tsp.	1 mL
Large egg	1	1
Milk	1 cup	250 mL
Canola oil	1/3 cup	75 mL

Heat first amount of canola oil in medium frying pan on medium. Add
onion and garlic. Cook for 5 to 10 minutes, stirring often, until onion is soft
and golden.

Combine flour and baking powder in large bowl.

Add onion mixture and next 5 ingredients. Stir. Make a well in centre.

Beat egg with fork in small bowl. Add milk and second amount of canola
oil. Stir. Add to well. Stir until just moistened. Grease 12 muffin cups with
cooking spray. Fill cups 3/4 full. Bake in 375°F (190°C) oven for 20 to
25 minutes until wooden pick inserted in centre of muffin comes out clean.
Let stand in pan for 5 minutes before removing to wire rack to cool. Makes
12 muffins.

*1 muffin: 200 Calories; 8.0 g Total Fat (3.9 g Mono, 1.9 g Poly, 1.2 g Sat); 22 mg Cholesterol;
25 g Carbohydrate; 1 g Fibre; 6 g Protein; 379 mg Sodium*

CHOICES: 1 Grains & Starches; 1 Vegetables; 1 Fats

Pictured on page 143.

Measurement Tables

Throughout this book measurements are given in Conventional and Metric measure. To compensate for differences between the two measurements due to rounding, a full metric measure is not always used. The cup used is the standard 8 fluid ounce. Temperature is given in degrees Fahrenheit and Celsius. Baking pan measurements are in inches and centimetres as well as quarts and litres. An exact metric conversion is given below as well as the working equivalent (Metric Standard Measure).

Spoons

Conventional Measure	Metric Exact Conversion Millilitre (mL)	Metric Standard Measure Millilitre (mL)
1/8 teaspoon (tsp.)	0.6 mL	0.5 mL
1/4 teaspoon (tsp.)	1.2 mL	1 mL
1/2 teaspoon (tsp.)	2.4 mL	2 mL
1 teaspoon (tsp.)	4.7 mL	5 mL
2 teaspoons (tsp.)	9.4 mL	10 mL
1 tablespoon (tbsp.)	14.2 mL	15 mL

Cups

Conventional Measure	Metric Exact Conversion Millilitre (mL)	Metric Standard Measure Millilitre (mL)
1/4 cup (4 tbsp.)	56.8 mL	60 mL
1/3 cup (5 1/3 tbsp.)	75.6 mL	75 mL
1/2 cup (8 tbsp.)	113.7 mL	125 mL
2/3 cup (10 2/3 tbsp.)	151.2 mL	150 mL
3/4 cup (12 tbsp.)	170.5 mL	175 mL
1 cup (16 tbsp.)	227.3 mL	250 mL
4 1/2 cups	1022.9 mL	1000 mL (1 L)

Oven Temperatures

Fahrenheit (°F)	Celsius (°C)
175°	80°
200°	95°
225°	110°
250°	120°
275°	140°
300°	150°
325°	160°
350°	175°
375°	190°
400°	205°
425°	220°
450°	230°
475°	240°
500°	260°

Dry Measurements

Conventional Measure Ounces (oz.)	Metric Exact Conversion Grams (g)	Metric Standard Measure Grams (g)
1 oz.	28.3 g	28 g
2 oz.	56.7 g	57 g
3 oz.	85.0 g	85 g
4 oz.	113.4 g	125 g
5 oz.	141.7 g	140 g
6 oz.	170.1 g	170 g
7 oz.	198.4 g	200 g
8 oz.	226.8 g	250 g
16 oz.	453.6 g	500 g
32 oz.	907.2 g	1000 g (1 kg)

Pans

Conventional Inches	Metric Centimetres
8x8 inch	20x20 cm
9x9 inch	23x23 cm
9x13 inch	23x33 cm
10x15 inch	25x38 cm
11x17 inch	28x43 cm
8x2 inch round	20x5 cm
9x2 inch round	23x5 cm
10x4 1/2 inch tube	25x11 cm
8x4x3 inch loaf	20x10x7.5 cm
9x5x3 inch loaf	23x12.5x7.5 cm

Casseroles

CANADA & BRITAIN		UNITED STATES	
Standard Size Casserole	Exact Metric Measure	Standard Size Casserole	Exact Metric Measure
1 qt. (5 cups)	1.13 L	1 qt. (4 cups)	900 mL
1 1/2 qts. (7 1/2 cups)	1.69 L	1 1/2 qts. (6 cups)	1.35 L
2 qts. (10 cups)	2.25 L	2 qts. (8 cups)	1.8 L
2 1/2 qts. (12 1/2 cups)	2.81 L	2 1/2 qts. (10 cups)	2.25 L
3 qts. (15 cups)	3.38 L	3 qts. (12 cups)	2.7 L
4 qts. (20 cups)	4.5 L	4 qts. (16 cups)	3.6 L
5 qts. (25 cups)	5.63 L	5 qts. (20 cups)	4.5 L

Recipe Index

154

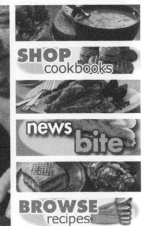

Cranberry Pistachio Cookies

Entertaining For The Holidays, Page 130

Butter, softened	1 cup	250 mL
Granulated sugar	1 cup	250 mL
Large egg	1	1
Egg yolk (large)	1	1
Grated orange zest	1 tbsp.	15 mL
Vanilla extract	1 tsp.	5 mL
All-purpose flour	2 1/2 cups	625 mL
Ground cinnamon	1/2 tsp.	2 mL
Ground allspice	1/4 tsp.	1 mL
Salt	1/4 tsp.	1 mL
Chopped dried cranberries	1 1/2 cups	375 mL
Chopped pistachios	1 1/2 cups	375 mL

Beat butter and sugar in large bowl until light and fluffy. Add next 4 ingredients. Beat well.

Combine next 4 ingredients in small bowl. Add to butter mixture in 2 additions, mixing well after each addition, until no dry flour remains.

Add cranberries and pistachios. Mix well. Divide into 2 portions. Roll into 9 inch (23 cm) long logs.

Wrap with plastic wrap. Chill for at least 6 hours or overnight. Cut into 1/4 inch (6 mm) slices with serrated knife. Arrange, about 2 inches (5 cm) apart, on greased cookie sheets. Bake in 375°F (190°C) oven for about 10 minutes until golden. Let stand on cookie sheets for 5 minutes before removing to wire racks to cool. Makes about 64 cookies.

1 cookie: 76 Calories; 4.4 g Total Fat (1.5 g Mono, 0.6 g Poly, 2.0 g Sat); 14 mg Cholesterol; 9 g Carbohydrate; 1 g Fibre; 1 g Protein; 43 mg Sodium

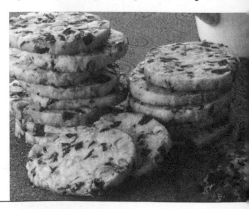

Celebrating the
Harvest
RECIPES FOR FALL & WINTER GATHERINGS

Whether from the garden, farmers' market or supermarket, harvest ingredients display the bounty and beauty of nature. Entertain a crowd in style, or feed your family comfort food they'll not soon forget—with new delicious recipes that celebrate harvest ingredients. What a lovely way to get through the long fall and winter!

SPECIAL OCCASION SERIES

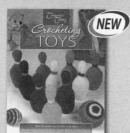 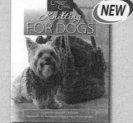 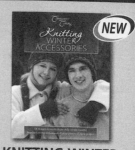
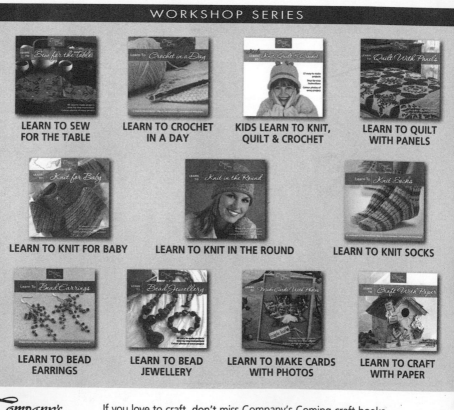
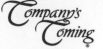